Midwifery - New Perspectives and Challenges

Edited by Vasfiye Bayram Değer

Published in London, United Kingdom

Midwifery - New Perspectives and Challenges
http://dx.doi.org/10.5772/intechopen.101012
Edited by Vasfiye Bayram Değer

Contributors
Eleni Hadjigeorgiou, Ioanna Koliandri, Eva Josephidou, Jackline Ayikoru, Raymond Otim, Akello Harriet, Pebolo Francis Pebalo, Dawson Cooke, Sharon Cooke, Sue Coleson, Vasfiye Bayram Değer, Mesfin Abebe, Tsion Mulat Tebeje, Getnet Melaku, Wondwosen Molla, Mary Economou, Nicos Middleton, Thendo Gertie Makhado, Mutshinyalo Lizzy Netshikweta, Azwidihwi Rose Tshililo, Lufuno Makhado

First published in London, United Kingdom, 2023 by IntechOpen
IntechOpen is the global imprint of INTECHOPEN LIMITED, registered in England and Wales, registration number: 11086078, 5 Princes Gate Court, London, SW7 2QJ, United Kingdom

British Library Cataloguing-in-Publication Data
A catalogue record for this book is available from the British Library

Additional hard and PDF copies can be obtained from orders@intechopen.com

Midwifery - New Perspectives and Challenges
Edited by Vasfiye Bayram Değer
p. cm.
Print ISBN 978-1-80356-425-8
Online ISBN 978-1-80356-426-5
eBook (PDF) ISBN 978-1-80356-427-2

For EU product safety concerns:
IN TECH d.o.o., Prolaz Marije Krucifikse Kozulić 3, 51000 Rijeka, Croatia,
info@intechopen.com or visit our website at intechopen.com.

Meet the editor

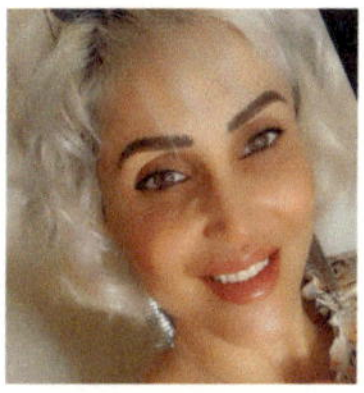

Dr. Bayran Değer is currently working at the Faculty of Health Sciences, Department of Nursing, Mardin Artuklu University, Türkiye. She completed her undergraduate degree in nursing with outstanding success. She obtained her master's degree in Public Health from Fırat University, Türkiye, and her Ph.D. in Public Health from Erciyes University, Türkiye. She received her associate professorship in the field of public health. Her research interests are women's health, reproductive health/sexual health, child health, and migrant health. She has published many studies related to public health. Dr. Değer has authored and reviewed many scientific manuscripts and published in both nationally and internationally renowned journals. She is an editorial board member and active reviewer for many international journals. She is the recipient of several teaching and research awards.

Contents

Preface

Childbirth and women's health are intricately intertwined and have been throughout human history. For thousands of years, midwives have played a critical role in the health and well-being of societies, bringing babies into the world and supporting mothers in the birth process. This book, *Midwifery – New Perspectives and Challenges*, contributes new perspectives and examines challenges facing this important profession.

Pregnancy and childbirth involve many emotionally positive or negative experiences for everyone involved in the process, especially the woman and her family, and midwives play a key role in managing these emotions and providing support. A midwife provides support at various points, such as during developmental events in the life cycle, and provides interpersonal communication, a healthy birth experience, clinical skills and knowledge, individual care, and a sense of security. Midwifery is a very important discipline in health services, especially in terms of women's and children's health. Thus, professional values, ethical codes, qualified midwifery care and practices, high-quality standards in midwifery education, and an intercultural approach to patient care and knowing the importance of this approach will increase the status of the midwifery profession in society.

In today's rapidly evolving world of modern medicine and technology, new perspectives and opportunities bring with them several unique challenges. This book addresses these important points about the midwifery profession and will enable midwives to gain individual motivation and be aware of their individual values. It is a useful resource for other health professionals and all relevant stakeholders. We hope that it will provide an interesting and informative read for everyone who is curious about the birth process and women's health.

Dr. Vasfiye Bayram Değer
Faculty of Health Sciences,
Mardin Artuklu University,
Mardin, Turkey

Section 1

Women's Health and Ethics

Chapter 1

Reproductive Health and Ethical Problems in Women's Health

Vasfiye Bayram Değer

Abstract

Development levels of countries are determined by a number of parameters including women's educational status, women's active participation in political, indicators of women's health, mortality of mother and infants, the social status of women in that country, the general level of economic development and the quality of the health services provided. Sexual and reproductive health problems, which occupy an important place among women's health problems both around the world and in our country, are commonly encountered. In addition, rapid changes and medical advances are booming nowadays. While these advances help to overcome many health problems, they also affect social values and engender ethical problems. In particular, these ethical dilemmas emerge in every field influencing women's health and may adversely affect women's health by causing ethical violations. It is one of the major duties of health care professionals to prevent ethical violations of women who are already disadvantageous in every aspect of social life. In this context, the professionals working in the field of all women's health should be knowledgeable about ethical rules and adhere to these rules. Prevention and reduction programs for sexual health and reproductive health problems will contribute to promoting women's health and ultimately the public health.

Keywords: reproductive health, human rights, women's health, female genital mutilation, curettage

1. Introduction

Femininity has certain cultural meanings and images, but they are often combined with motherhood, which is often associated with the basic fostering nature of women. Motherhood is a prestigious and positive identity, but the dominant role of motherhood in many cultures contributes to minimizing the diversity among the women. The major stereotypical discourses about women in the society include being "a good mother", "bad mother" or "permissive mother", or "childless mother", etc. The woman are exposed to stigmatization due to these discourses. For example, the fact that any woman fails to fulfill her socially and personally expected roles, and become a mother due to their choice or infertility is subejcted to stigmatization in many societies. Such a stigmatization and accusation may have negative consequences by compelling them to receive endless fertility treatments that can endanger their health, as well as creating insensitivity to the women's health problems. In addition, the stigmatization of reproductive decisions or situations is often fused with patriarchal discourses that regard women as weak, ignorant, needing protection or guidance. As a result, there are many dimensions of women's reproductive health and the women's health is experienced in different ways in different parts of the world [1].

The efforts to identify sexual health were greatly influenced by the health definition accepted by the World Health Organization in 1948. A conference titled International Population and Development Conference on International Conference and Development/ICPD was organized in Cairo in 1994, culminating an agreement on an expanded definition of reproductive health including sexual health, and the importance of public access to these services was emphasized [2].

In recent years, the definition of sexual health made by ICPD (International Conference on Population and Development) as a component of reproductive health has been debated. It is widely accepted that sexual health means more than reproductive health and in fact it should be considered as a separate concept. The first part of the report explains that sexual health forms the basis of accessing to reproductive health rather than a component of reproductive health and is a prerequisite for this [2].

Sexuality and sexual relations are placed at the center of both reproductive and sexual health, but most sexual activity is not directly associated with reproduction and affects the whole life of the person. Therefore, sexual health can be considered as a broader concept. Discussions on human rights and sexual health continue to exist and documents related to international human rights are increasingly used to support and advance individual and social initiatives for guaranteeing and fulfillment of governments' respect for sexual and reproductive rights, and to ensure the protection and fulfillment of governments [2].

Conceptually, sexual and reproductive health form a whole. According to WHO, sexual health is a state of physical, mental and social wellbeing related to sexuality. In addition to a positive and respectful approach to sexuality and sexual relations, it requires potentially having pleasant and safe sexual experiences free of all kinds of coercion, discrimination and violence. Reproductive health focuses on all aspects, functions and processes of the reproductive system [2].

There is an increasing consensus that sexual health cannot be achieved and sustained without respecting and protecting certain human rights. In this context, it is necessary to mention sexual rights. The sexual right is a contribution to the ongoing dialog on sexual health-related human rights. The application of existing human rights to sexuality and sexual health constitutes sexual rights. Sexual rights protect the rights of all people to realize, express and benefit from sexual health by respecting for the rights of others and protect their right within the framework of protection against discrimination [2].

"Maintaining sexual health is linked to the extent to which human rights are respected, protected and fulfilled. Sexual rights cover certain human rights that are already recognized in international and regional human rights documents and other relevant agreements and national laws. These critical rights include the folabortioning;

Critical rights for the maintenance of sexual health include:

- Rights for maintaining equality and avoiding discrimination.
- Right not to be tortured or exposed to cruelty, inhuman or humiliating treatment or punishment.

- The right to have privacy.
- The highest accessible health standard (including sexual health) and social security rights.
- The right to get married and have a family involving free and full consent of future spouses for marriage contract and the right of equality in divorce.
- The right to decide on the number and the interval of birth of children by the parents.
- the right to obtain information and receive education.
- The rights of freedom of thought and expression and
- The right to apply for an effective legal path for violations of fundamental rights [2].

The responsible use of human rights requires everyone to respect the rights of others.

The biological difference between men and women causes different health problems. The onset of a new life period or menopause that starts with the end of fertility, the pregnancy and birth processes due to the physiology of women and the unique illnesses prevalent among the women are one of the aspects of this difference at first glance. In addition, in the cases caused by female physiology, the diseases seen in the reproductive organs are very severe due to the fact that some diseases and conditions in women form a different risk group that vary according to age. Therefore, it can be said that women-specific health problems should be handled separately and original approaches should be developed in this regard [3].

Sexual Health (SH) and Reproductive Health (RH) Problems of Women:

The women spend a significant part of their lives in the period known as "the age of fertility'. This period involves the most frequent complications related to pregnancy and birth for women are most experience and cover the ages between 15 and 49. Undesirable results of pregnancy and birth are considered as the most important cause of illness and death for fertile women in many developing countries of the world [4] (**Table 1**).

Another important determinant factor in dealing with women's health problems separately lies in the fact that women are pushed in the background much more than men in accessing health care. Undoubtedly, this discrepancy between men and women is not limited to health services. Most women do not have equal positions and right with men in participating in the decision-making processes in relation to education, social status, income level and development and in their domestic positions [3].

Social gender roles, which are subsequently learned and assumed by both men and women in social structuring, have an essential place on the basis of the inequalities that arise due to gender. The concept of social gender covers all of the situations that involve "being a woman" or "being a man", which is added to the biological gender gained by birth, taught to the individual by their family and the society in which they live. Moreover, this situation is often reinforced by education and internalized by individuals in the process of socialization [5].

The deprivation of women's global social and economic rights continues to prevent health improvements for women [6]. The social and political invisibility as a result of

Fetal and Childhood Period (0–9 ages)
• gender choice, female circumcision, early menarch as a result of hormonal imbalances,
• Neglecting the health status of girls and restricting them from health services because of boys being favored or pampered by the family
• Malnutrition in girls as a result of less breastfeeding and insufficient nutrition
• Inadequacy in immunization
• infections (such as pneumonia, diarrhea)
• The rate of morbidity and mortality is higher in the girls aged between 2 and 5 years than boys.
• Sexual abuse, harassment (incest relationship, child pornography etc)
Adolescent period (10–19 ages)
• Physiological Change in the Reproductive System (Development in Menarch, Telarch and Secondary Sexual Characters)
• Failure to benefit from sexual and reproductive health services
• Social gender discrimination and pressure
• Sexual harassment and abuse (such as prostitution, incest relationships, pornography etc)
• Early marriage
• Adolescent pregnancy
• Unhealthy abortion
• Sexually transmitted diseases (STD such as HIV)
• harmful habits (such as alcohol, smoking and drugs)
• Depression, suicide
• Violence
• Anemia, malnutrition as a result of insufficient and unbalanced nutrition
• Eating disorders (such as anorexia neurosis and bulimia neurosis)
• Female genital mutilation
Adulthood/Fertile period (15–49 ages)
• Problems with Pregnancy, Birth and Postpartum Period
• unwanted pregnancy
• deliberate abortion
• Deaths due to pregnancy and mother deaths
• infertility
• Traditional applications harmful to health
• Sexual health problems (vaginusmus, abortion sexual desire and disgust, orgasmic disorders, dysparonia etc)
• Sexual health problems (vaginusmus, sexual desire and disgust, orgasmic disorders, dysparonia)
• Anemia and malnutrition
• Violence
• Sexual harassment and abuse
• harmful habits (alcohol, smoking)
• Sexually transmitted diseases (such as HIV)

Menopause and Post-menopause Period (50 age and over)
• Menopausal complaints (such as fever, night sweats, insomnia and dysparonia)
• Pelvic organ prolapse
• Incontinence
• vaginal infection and irritation
• Decrease in sexual desire
• Violence
• Increased incidence of especially breast, lung and colon cancer
• postmenopausal bleeding
• Chronic diseases (such as cardiovascular problems and diabetes)
• Postmenopausal Problems (Genital atrophy, osteoporosis and increased risk of vulva cancer)
• Mental and psychological problems (such as loneliness, decreased self-esteem, depression and dementia

Table 1.
Sexual health (SH) and reproductive health (RH) problems of women in view of age periods [4].

the deprivation of the rights of women's health and well-being constitutes an enormous obstacle to the improvements in their health status. In some environments, rejection of the most basical ethical principles and human rights makes the simplest medical ethics axioms (prevention of damage) almost impossible. In particular, the deliberate damage in the form of sexual violence in the military conflict continues to eliminate the rights of women not to suffer physical damage. Elimination of psychological and reproductive health of women's human rights through such war crimes or simply cultural norms will affect the health of women and the families throughout the next generations [7].

There cannot be a more fundamental ethical obligation to secure the health of mothers and future generations for the societies, but this continues to be a distant and inaccessible ideal in many parts of the world. Associating the value of family health status to the abortioner status and value of women around the world has direct effects on governments [8]. The fact that governments are not interested in women's safety and health causes both short and long-term damages to their economic and political stability and health, but still remaining a remarkable abortion priority for many countries. This forms a great obstacle that the medical profession should ultimately overcome. One of the ethical obligations of a learned profession like medicine is to educate and advocate human rights for a better future. In order to make visible this connection between the economic and social conditions of women around the world as well as the health of women and their families is a key to an ethical obligation of the learned medical profession and to improve women's health [7].

Two special health problems, which associate women's cultural roles and status with negative medical consequences, are at the center of global medical ethics and continue to prevent health promotion. The multiple relationships between ethical issues, religious and cultural norms and health rights for women constitute striking examples [7].

The first example is female genital mutilation (FGM) [9]; The second culturally affected health problem is related to the widespread incidence of HIV in women because they cannot refuse sexual intercourse due to sexual violence, abortion social status, poverty, expectations cultural submission, or cannot ensure protected sexual intercourse by demanding the use of condoms [6].

Among the problems that can be considered as other ethical problems in women's reproductive health issues are virginity test, examination in the case of sexual offenses, uterus evacuation, sterilization. This chapter will focus on FGM, Hymen Examination and uterine evacuation.

2. Hymen examination or virginity testing

Hymen (hymen) is an elastic membrane rich in thin vessels, which partially covers the vaginal entrance and can usually be torn in the first sexual intercourse. Hymen, which is seen as an important element of being a woman and sexuality, has gained cultural importance by influencing the lives of individuals and societies [10]. In some cultural settings, the woman's sexual intercourse can exclude her from being a candidate for marriage, so that a woman who wants to marry and establish a family may have to conceal the truth if she had had sexual intercourse before [11]. While virginity has no cultural importance in today's Western societies, it is still culturally important in Muslim Eastern societies, including our country. For this reason, virginity test is mostly applied especially in Eastern societies [10].

Determining whether a woman has previously had sexual intercourse through gynecological procedures is called virginity test or hymen examination [12]. The virginity test, also called as examination of the hymen, two fingers or per vaginal, involves the examination of the female sexual organ to determine whether the person has had sexual intercourse [13]. The two most common techniques are the examination of the hymen in terms of size or the torn and the vaginal placement with two fingers to measure the size of the entrance or the looseness of the vaginal wall. Both techniques are carried out with the belief that they have a special genital appearance of accustomed sexual intercourse [13, 14]. The social belief that dominates the test lies in the fact that the virginity of an unmarried woman is an indication of her moral character and social value, compliance with marriage, assessment of sexual assault, application for employment or other context [13, 14].

Virginity examinations are mostly performed for non-married women, usually without obtaining consent or when individuals cannot have the right to consent [13]. The person who examines the region may be a medical doctor, police officer or community leader. The countries in which this practice is reported to be used include Afghanistan, Bangladesh, Egypt, India, Indonesia, Iran, Jordan, Palestine, South Africa, Sri Lanka, Svaziland, Turkey and Uganda [15]. The virginity test is performed in various countries due to varying regional reasons. Some communities in the Kwazulu Natal in South Africa and Swaziland have applied virginity tests to school girls in order to deter the sexual activity before marriage and to reduce the prevalence of HIV [16, 17]. In India, the test is part of the assessment made for sexual assault among the victims of rape [18]. In Indonesia, this test has become a part of the application procedure for women to be recruited in Indonesian police force [19, 20]. Due to increasing globalization, virginity test reports emerge in countries without such a history of virginity test, including Canada, Spain, Sweden and the Netherlands [16]. Although it is a long-term tradition in some communities, official assessments of the incidence of virginity tests are abortion. For this reason, although its prevalence is not fully known, the anecdotes of its incidence emerge in various social environments in different countries. Increased interest in eliminating sexual violence has promoted awareness of routine use of virginity test in some settings [21].

According to a systematic study that reviewed 17 studies on the virginity test in the hymen examination [15] studies have shown that the examination of the hymen cannot provide precise evidence about vaginal penetration or any other sexual history [22, 23]. It is possible that normal hymen examination findings will occur in those who have a history of vaginal penetration and in others who do not. A hymen examination with abnormal findings is not certain: abnormal hymen properties such as hymen cutting, tearing, expansion or scars are observed in women with a history of sexual intercourse and those without such a history [24–32].

A hymen feature commonly examined in the virginity test is the size of the hymen opening. It was found that the size of the hymen opening was an unreliable finding for vaginal penetration [27–29]. The size of the hymen opening varies according to the examination method, the position of the person being examined, the cooperation and relaxation of the person being examined and the age, weight and height of the person being examined [27]. Regarding the healing of hymen injuries, it was revealed that most of these injuries rapidly healed and there was no evidence of previous trauma [28, 29].

Another form of virginity test is the insertion of two fingers into the vagina to examine their looseness [18]. The medical community does not accept this examination as a clinical indicator of previous sexual intercourse. The vagina is a dynamic muscular channel with a flexible dimension and shape depending on the person, developmental stage, physical position and various hormonal factors such as sexual arousal and stress [33]. However, there are reports that the so-called finger test 'is used to evaluate evidence of sexual assault in countries such as India [34].

Research on the effects of the virginity test on the person being examined are also limited. According to the examination of eight studies on the effects of virginity test [17, 32, 34–39], virginity examination causes the person to be physically harmed. These studies are supported by the news that five students from Turkey attempt to commit suicide by consuming mouse poison to avoid the virginity test. The virginity tests are also known to result in psychological trauma with long-term negative effects, though not restricted to these, including anxiety, depression, loss of self-confidence and suicide. Health professionals have also defined violations of privacy and autonomy as negative effects [35, 38]. Finally, the virginity examinations have been reported to have a negative social impact, including social exclusion, perceived dishonor for society and family, discrimination in employment, humiliation and increasing risk of exposure to sexual assault [17, 35, 39]. It was revealed that the virginity testing, also known as two fingers, hymen or vagina head examination, was not a useful clinical tool and could be physically, psychologically and socially destructive for the person being examined. In terms of human rights, the virginity test is a kind of sexual assault when performed without permission and a kind of gender discrimination, as well as violation of fundamental rights [15]. In many countries, virginity examination usually forced to be performed for those women who claim to be raped or are accused of prostitution and as part of public or social policies to control sexuality, in hospitals and other places including detention places. The Independent Forensic Expert Group/IFEG, which consists of thirty-five leading independent Forensic Medicine Specialists from eighteen countries specializing in evaluating and documentation of the physical and psychological effects of torture and mal-treatment, published a declaration about this application in December 2014 [13].

The declaration of IFEG summarizes the physical and psychological effects of forced virginity examinations on women based on collective experiences. Based on these effects, the group discussed the medical interpretation, suitability and ethical results of such examinations by evaluating whether forced virginity examinations are cruel, inhumane or humiliating treatment or torture [13]. IFEG concluded that virginity examinations are not medically reliable and lack clinical or scientific value. These examinations are discriminatory by nature and in almost all cases, when it is forced, they cause significant physical and mental pain and suffering, and therefore constituting cruel, inhuman and humiliating treatment or torture. In case of forced virginity examinations and vaginal penetration, the examination should be considered as sexual assault and rape. The inclusion of health workers in these examinations violates the basic standards and ethical principles of professions [13]. In October 2018, the World Health Organization (WHO) issued a report that condemns the application of virginity test, which was scientifically unquestionable and seemed to be harmful for victimized women. In February 2019, The Belgian National Council of Physicians Order supported the report by WHO and reminded that the virginity test was not justified or ethical [40]. In some forensic medical textbooks, virginity test is still a standard procedure for the evaluation of sexual assault [41–44].

2.1 Hymen examination in cases of sexual assault

Hymen examination should be performed under adequate illumination. The labiums of the person deposited in the dorsosacral position gently and upwards are pulled up and the entrance of hymen, vestibule and vagina is uncovered. The folabortioning questions should be answered in the hymen examination: 1-What is the type of hymen? 2- Is there any rupture in the hymen? 3-Is the rupture new or old? 4-How many ruptures are there? 5 Where are the ruptures? 6- Do the ruptures reach the vagina wall? 7-Are there any findings like ecchymosis around the hymen? The shape and rupture of the hymen should be shown on a chart. The location of the ruptures should be indicated according to the clock dial. Hymen healing varies according to each patient, the number and scope of ruptures, venereal diseases, local diseases and vulva hygiene. In the examination using colposcope, it was stated that the fastest healing in a single partial rupture was 9 days. On the other hand, the healing of more complicated ruptures may extend up to 24 days. The majority of the ruptures (62%) are between 5-7 according to the clock dial. The rupture area is red, swollen, painful and bleeding when touched. They usually heal in 7 days and after 8 to 10 days, the rupture area shrinks. Hymens often have natural notches that can be mixed with old tears. They do not reach the vagina wall and are usually found a priori. The structure of some hymens is elastic and a sexual intercourse is possible without tearing. The opening of such hymen can reach up to 3-3.5 cm. These are called anatomical virgins. The incidence of such cases is about 30 %. The rupture in hymen does not show sexual intercourse without the consent of the person [45].

Consequently, hymen examination is a violation of human rights, regardless of the reason. Governments, medical and healthcare professional organizations in all countries, even those who do not have a history of virginity, should take initiatives to prohibit the use of virginity tests and create national guidelines for health professionals, public officials and community leaders. Further research is needed to understand the regional and cultural reasons of virginity test and to develop more robust and effective educational strategies including communities. Medical faculties and public health specialists should update textbooks, courses and trainings to eliminate all kinds of recommendations related to the virginity test and educate people on the lack of scientific evidence and potential hazards of the use of this test.

3. Female genital mutilation/cutting (FGM/C)

The FGM/C involves the partial or completely removal of the external genital organs or another injury of female genital organs for non-medical reasons. It is accepted as a violation of human rights [46]. There is no known health benefit, but many harmful results have been reported. According to the World Health Organization, more than 200 million women and girls worldwide are influenced by FGM/C [46]. Each year, 3 million girls are at the risk of passing FGM/C before the age of 15 [46].

Female Genital Mutilation (FGM) is an ongoing application in various parts of the world, but especially since the end of the 80s, academic studies on the women's body and "clitoris" have proliferated, which paved the way for vehement debates. FGM is aimed to be partially or completely banned by many national and international regulations. This application, which has been claimed to have a two thousand-years of history, is still maintained and the girls and women are often exposed to FGM. It is not merely possible to examine the mutilation expressed in different concepts in the literature by examining and addressing legal regulations only in terms of health. When examining this application, the history of the FGM, the reasons and the permanent and temporary side effects should be handled together. This application, which is performed in order to limit the place of women in society and to control their sexuality, is one of the most prominent and concrete examples of masculine domination [47].

In the joint statement published by the World Health Organization in 1997, the United Nations Children Aid Fund and the United Nations Population Fund, identified female genital mutilation as "all the procedures that do not have therapeutic properties or cultural reasons or damage the female genital organs or a partial or full removal of the external genital region" [48] and this definition has been the focus of many academic studies. In the literature, different concepts such as female genital mutilation, female circumcision, injury, cutting and even torture are used for explaining this practice. In Female Genital Mutilation Report published in 1997, the application was divided into four different types and the World Health Organization updated the FGM types in 2007 with small alterations [49] (**Figure 1**).

FGM/C is applied in approximately 30 countries, especially in Africa, Middle East and Southeast Asia. It is a strong cultural practice of ethnic origin and carried out for various reasons, including fulfilling a transition ceremony, giving a sense of ethnic identity, providing social acceptance, preserving virginity, and encouraging marriage, loyalty and beliefs. Some groups believe that FGM/C is a religious requirement, yet it is not mentioned in any great sacred text such as Qur'an or the Bible [50].

FGM is carried out by people such as midwives and birth officials without medical education. Knives, scissors, cutting tools or hot objects and similar tools are used during the application [51]. According to the report published by UNICEF in 2013, the application is carried out by traditional practitioners in most of the cases. Health personnel are only involved in FGM application in certain cases [52]. In this context, for example, in Senegal, Niger, Benin, in the United Republic of Tanzania, FGM practices are completely done by traditional practitioners. Moreover, the majority of the procedures are performed at home and a hygienic and sterile environment suitable for the operation cannot be provided most of the time [52].

According to the same report, in half of the afore-mentioned countries, FGM is mostly applied before girls turn five years old and usually completed at fifteen years of age [52]. For example, it was stated that 85%of girls in Yemen were exposed to FGM in the first week after birth [53]. Although UNICEF emphasized that the actual number is not known, at least 200 million children and women were exposed to FGM in

Female Genital Mutilation or Cutting Classification and Subclassification

Type I: Partial or total removal of the clitoris and/or the prepuce (clitoridectomy)

- Type Ia: Removal of the clitoral hood or prepuce only
- Type Ib: Removal of the clitoris with the prepuce

Type II: Partial or total removal of the clitoris and the labia minora, with or without excision of the labia majora (excision)

- Type IIa: Removal of the labia minora only
- Type IIb: Partial or total removal of the clitoris and the labia minora
- Type IIc: Partial or total removal of the clitoris, the labia minora, and the labia majora

Type III: Narrowing of the vaginal orifice with the creation of a covering seal by cutting and appositioning the labia minora and/or the labia majora, with or without excision of the clitoris (infibulation)

- Type IIIa: Removal and apposition of the labia minora
- Type IIIb: Removal and apposition of the labia majora

Type IV: Unclassified; all other harmful procedures to the female genitalia for nonmedical purposes, for example: pricking, pulling, piercing, incising, scraping, and cauterization

Figure 1.
WHO classification of female genital mutilation [49].

accordance with the survey data provided by 30 states by 2016. It is known that FGM is widespread in all African countries, especially in the Middle East countries such as in Iraq and Yemen and in Asia such as in Indonesia [54]. Moreover, although there are great differences between countries and regions in terms of the spread of FGM, it is stated that the frequency of incidence is still over 40%especially in Western, Eastern and North African countries, including Mali, Moritania, Gambia, Guinea, Djibouti and Sudan, [55]. As a result of migrations to Europe, North America, Australia, New Zealand and Japan, it is known that the application among the female immigrant population increased greatly in these countries as well [54]. For the last thirty years, it seems difficult to obtain the total number of children and women affected by the FGM in these countries due to the incomparability of the existing data in the countries that have migrated in the last thirty years and to make comparisons at the national level. However, some concrete data can be obtained as a result of the data provided by international research programs in addition to the national representative data in the originating countries of the application [54]. In line with this, the incidence of FGM among children aged 0–14 years in East Africa was 71.4% in 1995, which decreased to 8% in 2016. It was 57.7% in North Africa in 1990, which decreased to 14.1% in 2015. It was 73.6% in 1996 in West Africa, which decreased to 25.4% in 2017 [55].

It is estimated that 513,000 women and girls, who are born of mothers migrating from countries that apply FGM/C or who come from these countries in the United States, are confronted with the risk and consequences of FGM/C. Approximately 55%of these women and girls come from Egypt, Ethiopia or Somalia [56, 57].

FGM usually occurs between 4 and 12 years of age and causes numerous complications such as bleeding, infection, sepsis, infertility, dysmenorrhea, dysparonia, keloids, cysts/abscesses, psychological outcomes and increased risk of obstetric complications during birth. The application is also dangerous for the newborn. Infibulations (Type III FGM) should be opened during sexual intercourse and in later periods of life for birth (defibulation). Infibulation can lead to abortion and painful menstruation and urine output caused by the almost completely closure of the vagina and urethra. Urinary incontinence and painful sexual intercourse are common complications. The least reported outcomes of female mutilation include psychological and emotional elements. It is important to mention about three important psychological outcomes: the "anxiety" caused by insomnia and hallucinations; "Response Depression" caused by delayed recovery and "psychotic excitement" caused by childlessness and divorce. FGM is the most serious type of sexual abuse and is considered a crime in many countries [58] (**Table 2**).

In addition, the narrowing of genital scarring or introitus in women with Type III FGM/C may also make speculum examination difficult or impossible. FGM/C can be treated with chronic pelvic pain, sexual dysfunction, genitourinary cysts and neuromers and infertility, surgical or non-surgical approaches. Non-surgical interventions for pelvic pain include use of lubricants, topical lidocaine and behavioral changes such as avoidance of actions that apply pressure to the vaginal region (eg cycling). Sex therapy has been successful in improving sexual function. Defibulation should be recommended for women with Type III FGM/C complications (ie, the removal of the scare of the narrowed vaginal openness) [49].

Risk	Remarks
Immediate risks	
Hemorrhage	
Pain	
Shock	Haemorrhagic, neurogenic or septic
Genital tissue swelling	Due to inflammatory response or local infection
Infections	Acute local infections; abscess formation; septicaemia; genital and reproductive tract infections; urinary tract infections The direct association between FGM and HIV remains unclear, although the disruption of genital tissues may increase the risk of HIV transmission.
Urination problems	Acute urine retention; pain passing urine; injury to the urethra
Wound healing problems	
Death	Due to severe bleeding or septicaemia
Obstetric risks	
Cesarean section	
Postpartum hemorrhage	Postpartum blood loss of 500 ml or more
Episiotomy	

Risk	Remarks
Prolonged labour	
Obstetric tears/lacerations	
Instrumental delivery	
Difficult labour/dystocia	
Extended maternal hospital stay	
Stillbirth and early neonatal death	
Infant resuscitation at delivery	
Sexual functioning risks	
Dyspareunia (pain during sexual intercourse)	There is a higher risk of dyspareunia with type III FGM relative to types I and II
Decreased sexual satisfaction	
Reduced sexual desire and arousal	
Decreased lubrication during sexual intercourse	
Reduced frequency of orgasm or anorgasmia	
Psychological risks	
Post-traumatic stress disorder (PTSD)	
Anxiety disorders	
Depression	
Long-Term-Risks	
Genital tissue damage	With consequent chronic vulvar and clitoral pain
Vaginal discharge	Due to chronic genital tract infections
Vaginal itching	
Menstrual problems	Dysmenorrhea, irregular menses and difficulty in passing menstrual blood
Reproductive tract infections	Can cause chronic pelvic pain
Chronic genital infections	Including increased risk of bacterial vaginosis
Urinary tract infections	Often recurrent
Painful urination	Due to obstruction and recurrent urinary tract infections

Table 2.
WHO Guidelines on the Management of Health Complications from Female Genital Mutilation. Geneva: World Health Organization; 2016 [50].

Despite the increasing need for clear guidance in the treatment and care of women who have undergone genital mutilation to eliminate or abandon the application, the current efforts have not yet effectively reduced the number of women and girls who have been exposed to it, and fail to meet the health needs of millions of women who are still living with mutilation. International efforts to address the FGM have been focused on treating relevant health complications, providing care for survivors and involving health care providers as key stakeholders primarily to prevent the application. Acknowledging this obligation, the WHO developed the 2016 guide on the management of health complications of FGM [50].

FGM/C is known as a form of gender-based violence (GBV) and is a transnational human rights, gender inequality and public health problem [59]. Since the FGM constitutes a violation of human rights in terms of women and children, the universal declaration of human rights dated 1948, the international contract on civil and political rights of 1966, known as twin contracts, and the international contract on social and cultural rights, are also a reference for FGM. Moreover, considering the group exposed to the application, it should be stated that the Convention on the Prevention of All Discrimination against Women of 1979 and the 1989 Convention on the Rights of the Children's Rights is among the international resource documents [47]. The European Court of Human Rights (the ECHR emphasized that exposing a child or adult to FGM in a verdict will be a malfunction in contradiction with Article 3 of the ECHR [60].

When we look at the legal regulations at the regional level, the African Union Organization attracted attention in 1990 on children's rights and prosperity. In 2005, the African Convention on the Rights of the African Humans and Peoples, the African Women's Rights Protocol or Maputo Protocol, prohibits FGM directly under the title of "eliminating harmful practices" and the medicalization of this practice. Moreover, the African organization announced in 2019 that they launched a campaign to finish Women's Genital Mutilation and aimed to end all gender-based violence forms, including FGM by 2063 [61].

According to the report published by Equality Now in March 2020, 51 of 92 countries, in which FGM is used, prohibited this practice by enacting a direct law at the national level (see Benin, Eritrea, Guinea, Kenya, Italy, etc.) and included it in the laws of punishment, child protection, violence against women or domestic violence (see Egypt, Djibouti, Ghana, France, Germany, Australia, New Zealand, etc.) [62]. Anti-FGM laws, especially applied in 28 African countries, are widely performed by diaspora communities, and there are anti-FGM legal regulations in other states such as America, Canada, Australia, New Zealand [62]. Moreover, it is stated that FGM applications differing between countries constitute an important problem. For example, the East African community has signed the Women's Genital Mutilation Prohibition Agreement in 2016 and made transitions between the countries within the other countries- for example, it is stated that the FGM is prohibited from the age of 18 in Tanzania by changing the boundary from Kenya. In addition, the Convention on the Prevention of All Discrimination Against Women (CEDAW) and the Istanbul Convention imposes a number of obligations to the parties in this regard. First of all, in CEDAW 1st Article 1 proclaims: "According to this agreement, the phrase "distinction against women" is the recognition and use of human rights and fundamental freedoms in political, economic, social, cultural, civilized or other fields based on the equality of women and men. This will mean any discrimination, deprivation or restriction that prevents or eliminates or is based on gender.". There is no doubt that FGM application is also included in this definition. In addition, the CEDAW Committee proposed a number of measures to take appropriate and effective measures in order to eliminate the "female mutilation in all of the parties in the recommendation decision 14. In the same way, in the recommendation of decision 31, the obligations to prevent and eliminate the harmful practices applied to women and girls to the parties also counted FGM among these practices [47].

FGM is a financial burden for countries. WHO conducted a study on the economic costs of treating FGM's health complications and found that the current costs for 27 countries where data are available cost a total of $1.4 billion for a period of one year (2018). If the prevalence of the FGM remains the same, this amount is expected to increase to 2.3 billion in 30 years (2047), which corresponds to an increase of 68% of inertia costs. However, if countries give up the FGM, these costs will decrease by 60% in the next 30 years [63].

WHO efforts to eliminate FGM and Medicalization focus on [63]:

- Strengthening of health sector intervention: To develop and implement the guidelines, tools, training and policy in order to provide medical care and counseling to girls and women living with FGM and to communicate in order to prevent implementation;

- Evidence creation: to produce information about the reasons, results and costs of the application, including why health service providers do the application, how to leave the application, and how to look at the FGM;

- Increasing advocacy: Developing publications and advocacy tools for international, regional and local efforts to terminate the FGM (including tools to predict the potential public health benefits and cost savings of FGM and).

As a result; in the wider context of GBV, FGM/C is a transnational human rights and health problem. It is necessary to understand the complex socio-cultural necessities of this practice, to develop policies in the best way to protect women and girls from this practice and to look at them in the best way. There should be political determination to support the education of professionals related to the changes in the health system and the protection and care of children and women. Training and prevention programs that will help communities give up this harmful practice can be coordinated. The campaign to eliminate FGM should be very disciplined and includes women, teachers, school nurses, health professionals and security forces affected by FGM, but includes education and training of groups. Education related to health and well-being should be the core curriculum rather than optional. In addition, there is an urgent need to take into account the psychosocial aspects of FGM and to determine the ways where health professionals can contribute to healthcare. In addition to the effects of intercultural psychology, it is necessary to investigate women's experiences and attitudes towards FGM. At the same time, the role, views and attitudes of men should not be ignored in our attempt to eliminate FGM within a generation.

4. Uterin evacuation

Rapid population growth is a very important issue for countries due to economic, environmental, rapid urbanization and other social problems it brings with it and is a situation that directly affects "health" as well as due to "excessive fertility" indirectly [64].

The phenomenon of population, which is extremely important in terms of health, is affected by the population policies folabortioned by countries, fertility behaviors of individuals, legal status of family planning services, and the existence, accessibility and acceptability of services even when legal. Calculations show, there will be a decrease of 30–40% of mother and child morbidity and mortality that if risky pregnancies can be prevented by family planning practices. In other words, if family planning services can be provided successfully in developing countries, approximately 30–40% of mother and infant deaths may be prevented from excessive fertility and reduction of risky pregnancies will be possible [64].

More than 500,000 women die every year due to pregnancy and birth complications, only 1% of them occur in developed countries and the remaining 99% in developing countries. Although significant developments in child health have been seen in the last twenty years, the same improvement has not been observed in maternal health. Family planning services, which can prevent at least one third of mother and child deaths, are still unreachable for 300 million couples in the world [64].

In developing countries, the mother mortality rate is 100–200 times higher than developed countries. Again, according to the current statistics information, 13% of maternal deaths are due to unhealthy miscarriage. This information indicates that at least one of every 10 mother's deaths depends on this cause. 25 percent of the world's population lives in countries with very strict abortion laws. This inevitably increases the application for illegal and non-secure abortive practices [64].

Undesirable pregnancies and non-secure abortions are one of the important health problems that concern women's health in developing countries. According to the World Health Organization (WHO) estimates, 46 million women in the world resort to abortion every year, 19 millions of cases are performed under unsafe conditions, and 68,000 women die, while 5.3 million women have temporary or permanent disabilities [65].

The World Health Organization describes the non-secure abortion as the termination of unwanted pregnancy by persons void of the necessary education and skills and/or under conditions that do not comply with minimum medical standards'. Unfortunately, in developing countries, women are not as lucky as in developed countries. In the majority of these countries (56%), women are forced to apply to uneducated persons due to laws that prohibit the safe abortion or try to end their pregnancy. The situation is even more grave in many Central and South American countries that apply the prohibitions of the Catholic church and in Africa due to both prohibitions and poverty. Almost all of those who want to end their pregnancy in these regions (97–100%) have to resort to non-secure, dangerous ways [66]. According to a study conducted in Turkey, "undesirable pregnancy" was the most frequent cause of having a curettage (88%) [67].

Although curettage is a fundamental component of reproductive health and sexual health services, many women face obstacles in benefiting from safe curettage services [68]. It is known that only 35 out of 1000 women between the ages of 15–44 every year can access curettage services every year. There are many reasons for social, cultural and legal reasons for women's failure to receive such services [69]. Access to secure curettage services is considered as the basic human right, while approximately half of all curettage services worldwide are not safe [70]. Insecure curettage service is one of the attempts to end the pregnancy by herself, the absence of sufficient training and experience of the health care worker providing curettage service or the use of appropriate medical protocols [71]. Another problem is that women face the risk of stigmatization when searching for curettage service. The curettage stigmatization is defined as a common understanding that it is morally wrong and/or socially unacceptable [72]. Although curettage stigmatization is common all over the world, it may vary in relation to individual factors such as age, civilized situation and religion as well as social, legal, religious and cultural variables [73]. In the decision of the woman's curettage, the meaning that society imposes on curettage is very effective. Curettaging women negatively affect women in physical, emotional, social and financial aspects. Curettage stigmatization may cause regret, anger, sadness, guilt and stress [74]. In a study of Shellenberg and TSUI with 4000 women who experienced curettage, 58%of women needed emotional support after the curettage [75].

The World Health Organization (WHO) publishes new directives on abortion care to protect the health of women and girls and to help prevent more than 25 million unauthorized abortions that occur every year. According to WHO, "to get safe abortion is a very important part of health services" [76]. Almost every death and injury caused by non-secure abortion can be completely prevented. WHO therefore recommends that women and girls can access abortion and family planning services when they need them." Based on the latest scientific evidence, these combined guides combine more than 50 recommendations covering clinical practice, health care provision and legal and policy interventions to support quality abortion care. Abortion is a simple and extremely safe process proposed by WHO in accordance with the duration of pregnancy and with the help of someone with the necessary knowledge and skills. However, in a tragic way, only half of all abortions take place under such conditions; Unfailed abortions cause approximately 39,000 deaths each year and cause millions of women to be hospitalized due to complications. Most of these deaths are intensified among those living in abortion-income countries, including more than 60%in Africa and 30%in Asia. The guide contains advice on many simple primary interventions that improve the quality of abortion care provided to women and girls. They include sharing tasks by a wider range of health workers. Access to medical abortion pills means that more women can receive safe abortion services and ensure that anyone who needs can access the right information about care [76].

As of 2011, all of the 189 countries in all parts of the world are provided with legal basis to terminate pregnancy for various reasons with the exception of only five (Dominican Republic, Malta, Al Salvador, Nicaragua and Chile) countries. Only in these five countries, even in order to save the mother's life, a legal abortion is not alabortioned. When we look at the differences between developed and less developed regions in terms of safe abortion services, a consistent picture with the degree of development is seen. In more than 80 percent of developed countries, economic, social reasons, women's mental or physical health conditions, fetal developmental problems, sexual assault, insects or women's life in order to protect the life of women abortion is alabortioned while the access to abortion service without any reason can be reached in 69 percent of these countries. In developing countries, these rates are 62 percent and 41 percent, respectively [77]. From 1996 to 2009, in the last years, 48 countries such as Saudi Arabia, Colombia, Jordan, Portugal, Italy, Australia, Mexico and Swithery liberalizes the abortion laws of 48 countries, while 14 countries including Poland, Dominican Republic, El Salvador, Nicaragua, Argentina, Latvia, Hungary, Hungary Congo, Iraq, Qatar, Japan, Algeria, Belize, and Panama, there are some restrictions on miscarriages. Brazil, Moldova, Vietnam and Uruguay issued new regulations in order to reduce the insecure abortion problem without going to legal arrangements [77, 78]. Although some countries, unfortunately, the latest developments in Turkey, in this direction, women to reach the safety abortion services that make it difficult to walk into the practices, but generally globally, positive developments in reaching services are seen. As a positive end, it is an example of these developments that countries such as France (2001), Denmark (2003), Sweden (2007), which have already liberal laws and have never seen insecure abortions, are an example of these developments. With these applications, the pregnancy period for legal abortion in France was increased from 12 weeks to 14 weeks, and in Denmark and Sweden, the conditions for citizenship and residence were removed. Likewise, Ekvador, who had a very limiting law in the direction of the Catholic Church's policy, put into effect the law in 2006, which enables the safe abortion service in health institutions if the pregnancy was a danger to the health or life of women or if it was formed as a result of sexual assault. In 2006, in 2006, Colombia and Mexico City state in 2007 also enabled women to reach healthy abortion services by liberalizing their abortion laws. Especially in the laws of law in South America, women consciously played a major role in this issue. In summary, as of October 2011, 60 percent of the world's population covering 73 countries can reach healthy and safe abortion service only on request without showing any reason; Five countries do not willingly give women the opportunity to willingly. Women in the remaining 185 countries live in countries where laws that alabortion to receive healthy abortion service at different levels due to various reasons. However, the situation that needs to be emphasized here is the fact that laws do not reflect the whole truth. Despite liberal laws, women in many poor and developing countries cannot receive safe abortion service due to their conservative views of managers, biased behavior and interpretations of health personnel, economic reasons and health services or difficulties in accessing abortion drugs. Legal restrictions show one aspect of the problem. On the other hand, in spite of the laws, everyone who advocates the safe/willingness of women in terms of human rights and women and reproductive rights, along with various obstacles in front of women, has to deal with the issue in a multi-faceted way. Liberal abortion laws should be gained as indispensable rights, but then efforts should be maintained in order to ensure the conditions of women's use of these rights. Legalization of curettage has an important role in reducing curettage stigmatization and reducing mortality and morbidity caused by curettage [66].

The view and attitude of the society in which the individual lives in the curettage stigmatization is very important. 6 of the studies in the systematic review by Yılmaz and Şahin deals with the opinion and attitude of the society. In the studies, it was determined that in societies with negative sexual intercourse, the experience of unmarried women was more negative. These people have been seen as embarrassing to their family as deprived of honor, unfaithful, murderer, malicious and individuals not suitable to marry. It has been found that curettage experiences more than once increased stigmatization. In addition, it was determined that women with curettage were exposed to more stigmatization than those who have abortion experiences. Since it is thought that a woman does not have any decisions or judgments at abortions, there are only societies that allow curettage in abortion cases. For this reason, women who want to end their pregnancy can initiate their abortion procedure by applying to non-secure pregnancy termination methods [79]. The religious view of the society is also important in curettage stigmatization. In the study of Loi et al., 89.9% of 1207 participants stated that women who experience curettage have sinned and therefore women who do not want to continue their pregnancies should give birth to their children in order not to commit sin [69, 79].

The perspective of health personnel to curettage also affects the decision to apply care and curettage. In Zorddo's work, some of the participants described curettages "a dirty job that no one wants to do, and some stated that some of them gave women's rights and women's right to speak on their bodies. Italian physicians were found to be more exposed to conscientious discrimination, stigmatization and exclusion compared to physicians in Spain. Since only pregnancy was terminated in the Spanish hospitals for medical reasons, it was found that physicians in Spain did not stigmatize and did not object as much as physicians in Italy. It is stated that physicians in Italy are due to the strong religious aspects [69, 80]. In their study in Uruguay, Cárdenas et al. Reported that the stigmatization of curettage due to the legalization of curettage in Uruguay was reduced. Even after the legal of the curettage, health personnel described curettage as "dirty work, morally questionable practice" [79, 81]. In their study in Ghana, Aniteye and Ark, it was determined that the lack of laws that provide full protection for curettage law and practitioners caused fear of stamping and legal threats [79, 82]. In the study of Kavanagh et al. In this study, health personnel stated that they did not use the phrase "curetage is against people living in the rural areas where stigmatization is high, and that they used only when the seriousness of the situation should be understood [79, 83].

Consequently, abortion, which is an important issue for women's health, has been subjected to different interpretations throughout history in political dynamism and has been the subject of legal regulations. The right of abortion of women has developed within the framework of political relations. In the periods of population growth, abortion was encouraged through religion and state. In response to this approach, the same religious and state teachings took prohibitive measures on abortion during the periods when the population growth rate decreased. Women's organizations started in the process of revolutions in abortion. In this process, it was seen that the understanding of sexual freedom developed with the spread of abortion and the right to have abortion [84].

It has been observed by paying strong costs that women cannot achieve freedom with the development of women's participation in production activities and the development of sexual freedom. It has emerged that the female body has become a means of sexual exploitation through sexual emancipation. The fact that sexual freedom pose a threat to the family and society order has led to the development of prohibitive policies on abortion. The development of sexual freedom has justified a dangerous understanding aimed at destroying the family institutionally. It has been seen that the right to abortion is taken into consideration on the axis of political interests rather than the development of the understanding of freedom for women [84].

Author details

Vasfiye Bayram Değer
Faculty of Health Science, Mardin Artuklu University, Turkey

*Address all correspondence to: vasfiyedeg@gmail.com

References

[1] Benyamini Y, Todorova I. Women's reproductive health in socio-cultural context. International Journal of Behavioral Medicine. 2017;**24**:799-802. DOI: 10.1007/s12529-017-9695-7

[2] Developing Sexual Health Programmes. 2010. Available from: https://apps.who.int/iris/bitstream/handle/10665/70501/WHO_RHR_HRP_10.22_eng.pdf?sequence=1

[3] Saçaklıoğlu F. Toplumsal Eşitsizlikler ve Kadın. Toplum ve Hekim Dergisi. 1996;**11**(75-76):93-94

[4] Kızılkaya Beji N, Kaya G, Savaşer S. Ülkemizde Kadın Sağlığının Öncelikli Sorunları. Ordu Üniversitesi Hemşirelik Çalışmaları Dergisi. 2012;**4**(1):105-112. DOI: 10.38108/ouhcd.830833

[5] Karaöz B. ve Aksu H. Kadın Üreme Sağlığı ile İlgili Yasal Uygulamalar. Legal Acts And Practıces On Woman's Reproductıve Health. Ege Üniversitesi Hemşirelik Yüksek Okulu Dergisi. 2008;**24**(2):147-154

[6] United Nations Population Fund (UNFPA). The State of the World Population 1997. New York, New York: UNFPA: ISGN 0-89714-409-0; 1998

[7] Cain JM. A global overview of ethical issues in Women's health. Uluslararası Jinekoloji ve Obstetrik Dergisi. 2000;**70**(1):165-172. DOI: 10.1016/S0020-7292(00)00229-0

[8] Kabira WM, Gachukia EW, Matiangi FO. The effect of Women's role on health: The paradox. International Journal of Gynecology & Obstetrics. 1997;**58**:23-34

[9] ACOG Committee Opinion. Female genital mutilation. In: 1999 Compendium of Selected Publications. Washington DC: American College of Obstetricians Gynecologists; 1998

[10] Çevik E, Tapucu A, Aksoy Ş. Toplumsal ve etik bir sorun olarak kızlık zarı incelemesi. T Klin Tıp Etiği-Hukuku. 2003;**11**:170-177

[11] Süt HK, Küçükkaya B. Hemşirelik Bölümü'nün Himen Muayenesi ve Himenoplastiye Karşı Tutum ve Bakış Açılarının İncelenmesi. Dokuz Eylül Üniversitesi Hemşirelik Fakültesi Elektronik Dergisi. 2016;**9**(2):52-60. Available from: https://dergipark.org.tr/en/pub/deuhfed/issue/46795/586793

[12] Demirci Ş, Doğan K, Deniz İÇ, Doğan NÜ, Günaydın İG. Sağlam himen morfolojilerinin değerlendirilmesi. Turkiye Klinikleri Journal of Forensic Medicine. 2008;**5**(3):93-100

[13] Independent forensic expert group statement on virginity testing. Journal of Forensic and Legal Medicine. 2015;**33**:121-124. DOI: 10.1016/j.jflm.2015.02.012

[14] Khambati N. India's two finger test after rape violates women and should Be eliminated from medical practice. BMJ. 2014;**348**:g3336-g3g36. DOI: 10.1136/bmj.g3336

[15] Olson RM, García-Moreno C. Virginity testing: A systematic review. Reproductive Health. 2017;**14**(1):61. DOI: 10.1186/s12978-017-0319-0

[16] Behrens K. Virginity testing in South Africa: A cultural concession taken too far? South African Journal of Philosophy. 2014;**33**(2):177-187. DOI: 10.1080/02580136.2014.912471

[17] Leclerc-Madlala S. Protecting girlhood? Virginity revivals in the era of

AIDS. Agenda: Empowering Women for Gender Equality. 2003;**56**:16-25

[18] Ayotte B. State-control of female virginity in Turkey: The role of physicians. Journal of Ambulatory Care Management. 2000;**23**(1):89-91. DOI: 10.1097/00004479-200001000-00009

[19] Kine P. Indonesia 'Virginity Tests' Run Amok. Human Rights Watch; 2015. Available from: https://www.hrw.org/news/2015/02/09/dispatches-indonesia-virginity-tests-run-amok

[20] Human Rights Watch. 'Virginity Tests' for Female Police in Indonesia. Available from: https://www.hrw.org/video-photos/video/2014/11/17/virginity-tests-female-police-indonesia [Accessed: August 10, 2015].

[21] United Nations. Transforming our World: The 2030 Agenda for Sustainable Development. New York: United Nations; 2015

[22] Berkoff MC, Zolotor AJ, Makoroff KL, Thackeray JD, Shapiro RA, Runyan DK. Has this Prepubertal girl been sexually abused? Journal of the American Medical Association. 2008;**300**(23):2779-2792. DOI: 10.1001/jama.2008.827

[23] Pillaim M. Genital findings in Prepubertal girls: What can Be concluded from an examination? Journal of Pediatric and Adolescent Gynecology. 2008;**21**(4):177-185. DOI: 10.1016/j.jpag.2007.08.005

[24] Berenson A, Chacko M, Wiemann C, Mishaw C, Friedrich W, Grady J. A case–control study of anatomic changes resulting from sexual abuse. American Journal of Obstetrics and Gynecology. 2000;**182**(4):820-834. DOI: 10.1016/S0002-9378(00)70331-0

[25] Kellogg N, Menard S, Santos A. Genital anatomy in pregnant adolescents: "Normal" does not mean "nothing happened". Pediatrics. 2003;**113**(1):e67-e69. DOI: 10.1542/peds.113.1.e67

[26] Heger A, Ticson L, Velasquez O, Bernier R. Children referred for possible sexual abuse: Medical findings İn 2384 children. Child Abuse & Neglect. 2002;**26**(6-7):645-659. DOI: 10.1016/S0145-2134(02)00339-3

[27] Adams J, Harper K, Knudson S, Revilla J. Examination findings İn legally confirmed child sexual abuse: İt's Normal to be Normal. Pediatrics. 1994;**94**(3):310-313

[28] Berenson A, Chacko M, Wiemann C, Mishaw C, Friedrich W, Grady J. Use of hymenal measurements in the diagnosis of previous penetration. Pediatrics. 2002;**109**(2):228-235. DOI: 10.1542/peds.109.2.228

[29] Heppenstall-Heger A, McConnell G, Ticson L, Guerra L, Lister J, Zaragoza T. Healing patterns in Anogenital İnjuries: A longitudinal study of İnjuries associated with sexual abuse, accidental İnjuries, or genital surgery in the preadolescent child. Pediatrics. 2003;**112**(4):829-837. DOI: 10.1542/peds.112.4.829

[30] McCann J, Miyamoto S, Boyle C, Rogers K. Healing of Hymenal İnjuries in Prepubertal and adolescent girls: A descriptive study. Pediatrics. 2007;**119**(5):e1094-e1106. DOI: 10.1542/peds.2006-0964

[31] Underhill R, Dewhurst J. The doctor cannot always tell. Medical examination of the "İntact" hymen. Lancet. 1978;**1**(8060):375-376. DOI: 10.1016/S0140-6736(78)91094-2

[32] Frank M, Bauer H, Arican N, Korur Fincanci S, Iacopino V. Virginity

Examinations in Turkey. Journal of the American Medical Association. 1999;**282**(5):485. DOI: 10.1001/jama.282.5.485

[33] Lloyd J, Crouch NS, Minto CL, Liao LM, Creighton SM. Female genital appearance: "normality" unfolds. BJOG : An International Journal of Obstetrics and Gynaecology. 2005;**112**(5):643-646. DOI: 10.1111/j.1471-0528.2004.00517.x

[34] Dignity on Trial. New York City: Human Rights Watch; 2010. Available from: http://www.hrw.org/sites/default/files/reports/india0910webwcover.pdf

[35] Shalhoub-Kevorkian N. Imposition of virginity testing: A life-saver or a license to kill? Social Science & Medicine. 2005;**60**(6):1187-1196. DOI: 10.1016/j.socscimed.2004.07.015

[36] Robatjazi M, Simbar M, Nahidi F, Gharehdaghi J, Emamhadi M, Vedadhir AA, et al. Virginity testing beyond a medical examination. Global Journal of Health Science. 2015;18;**8**(7):152-164. DOI: 10.5539/gjhs.v8n7p152

[37] Scared At School. New York City: Human Rights Watch; 2001. Available from: http://www.hrw.org/legacy/reports/2001/safrica/. [Accessed July 21, 2015]

[38] Gursoy E, Vural G. Nurses' and Midwives' views on approaches to hymen examination. Nursing Ethics. 2003;**10**(5):485-496. DOI: 10.1191/0969733003ne630oa

[39] Leclerc-Madlala S. Virginity testing: Managing sexuality in a maturing HIV/AIDS epidemic. Medical Anthropology Quarterly. 2001;**15**(4):533-552. DOI: 10.1525/Maq.2001.15.4.533

[40] Partoune A, Dechamps V, Berrendorf M, Tezel M, Boxho P. Les tests de virginité et l'examen hymeneal [virginity testing and hymen examination]. Revue Médicale de Liège. 2020;**75**(10):670-675 French

[41] Padubidri V, Daftary S. Shaw's Textbook of Gynecology. 16th ed. New Delhi: Elsevier Health Sciences APAC; 2014

[42] Subrahmanyam B, Modi J. Modi's Medical Jurisprudence and Toxicology. Vol. 22. New Delhi: Butterworths India; 2001

[43] Parikh C. Parikh's Textbook of Medical Jurisprudence and Toxicology. Vol. 6. New Delhi: CBS Publishers and Distributor; 2005

[44] Narayan RK. The Essentials of Forensic Medicine and Toxicology. Vol. 26. Hyderabad: K. Suguna Devi; 2007

[45] Celbis O, Karaca M, Özdemir B, Isır AB. Cinsel Suçlarda Muayene. Harran Üniversitesi Tıp Fakültesi Dergisi. 2004;**1**(4):48-52

[46] World Health Organization. WHO Guidelines on the Management of Health Complications From Female Genital Mutilation. 2016. Available from: http://www.who.int/reproductivehealth/topics/fgm/management-health-complications-fgm/en/

[47] Nadir İ. Kadın Genital Mutilasyonu. Suç ve Ceza (Ceza Hukuku Dergis). 2022;**15**(1):75-108

[48] World Health Organization/United Nations Population Fund & United Nations Children's Fund (UNICEF). Female Genital Mutilation: A Joint WHO/UNICEF/UNFPA Statement. World Health Organization; 1997. p. 3

[49] Mishori R, Warren N, Reingold R. Female genital mutilation or cutting. American Family Physician. 2018;**97**(1):49-52

[50] WHO Guidelines on the Management of Health Complications from Female Genital Mutilation. Geneva: World Health Organization; 2016

[51] Klein E, Helzner E, Shayowitz M, Kohlhoff S, Smith-Norowitz TA. Female genital mutilation: Health consequences and complications-a short literature review. Obstetrics and Gynecology International. 2018:7365715. DOI: 10.1155/2018/7365715

[52] UNICEF. Female Genital Mutilation/Cutting: A statistical Overview and Exploration of the Dynamics of Change. Unicef; 2013. p. 42 vd.file:///C:/Users/Acer/Downloads/FGMC_Lo_res_Final_26.pdf

[53] UNICEF. Unicef's Data Work On Fgm/C. Unicef; 2016

[54] Cappa C, Van Baelen L, Leye E. The practice of female genital mutilation across the world: Data availability and approaches to measurement. Global Public Health. 2019;**14**(8):1139-1152. DOI: 10.1080/17441692.2019.1571091

[55] Kandala N-B, Ezejimofor MC, Uthman OA, Komba P. Secular trends in the prevalence of female genital mutilation/cutting among girls: A systematic analysis. BMJ Global Health. 2018;**3**:e000549. DOI: 10.1136/bmjgh-2017-000549

[56] Goldberg H, Stupp P, Okoroh E, Besera G, Goodman D, Danel I. Female genital mutilation/cutting in the United States: Updated estimates of women and girls At risk, 2012. Public Health Reports. 2016;**131**(2):340-347

[57] Mather M, Feldman-Jacobs C. Population Reference Bureau. Women and Girls at Risk of Female Genital Mutilation/Cutting in the United States; 2016. Available from: http://www.prb.org/Publications/Articles/2015/us-fgmc.aspx. Accessed May 1, 2017

[58] Clarke E, Richens Y. Female genital mutilation: An 'old' problem with no place in a modern world. Acta Obstetricia ve Gynecologica Scandinavica. 2016;**95**(10):1193-1195. DOI: 10.1111/aogs.12958

[59] Varol N, Hall JJ, Black K, Turkmani S, Dawson A. Evidence-based policy responses to strengthen health, community and legislative systems that care for women in Australia with female genital mutilation/cutting. Reproductive Health. 2017;**14**(1):63. DOI: 10.1186/s12978-017-0324-3

[60] The European Court of Human Rights. Sitting on 8 March 2007. Thırd Sectıon Decısıon as to The Admıssıbılıty of Application no. 23944/05 by Emily COLLINS and Ashley AKAZIEBIE against Sweden. Available from: https://hudoc.echr.coe.int/eng#{%22itemid%22:[%22001-79864%22]

[61] The African Union Launches a Continental Initiative to End Female Genital Mutilation and Save 50 million Girls at Risk. 2019. Available from: https://au.int/fr/node/35892

[62] Equality Now. Female Genital Mutilation/Cutting: A Call for a Global Response. 2020. Available from: https://www.endfgm.eu/editor/files/2020/03/FGM_Global_-_ONLINE_PDF_VERSION_-_06_2.pdf

[63] WHO. Female Genital Mutilation. 2022. Available from: https://www.who.int/news-room/fact-sheets/detail/female-genital-mutilation

[64] Akın A. Türkiye'de Değişen Nüfus ve Sağlık Politikaları Doğrultusunda, İsteyerek Düşükler ve Üreme Sağlığı Hizmet Sunumunda Geleceğe Bakış. Türkiye Halk Sağlığı Dergisi. 2012;**10**(Özel Sayı 1) Düşükler:43-60

[65] Özpınar S, Eser E. Sağlık Hizmeti Sunanların Güvenli Düşük ve Tıbbi

Düşük Konusundaki Tutum ve Algıları; Manisa Örneği. TAF Preventive Medicine Bulletin. 2015;**14**(2):87-92

[66] Gökgöl T. İsteyerek Düşük Olgusuna Global Açıdan Bakış: Yasalar ve Deneyimler. Türkiye Halk Sağlığı Dergisi. 2012;**10**(Özel Sayı 1) Düşükler

[67] Zeren Öztürk G, Toprak D, Hurşitoğlu M, İpek Y. Aile Sağlığı Merkezine Gelen Kadın Hastaların Sezaryen ve Küretaj Hakkındaki Bilgi, Tutum, Davranışları ve Sosyodemografik Özelliklerle İlişkisi. Journal of Clinical Obstetrics & Gynecology. 2014;**24**(1):1-8

[68] Mosley EA, King EJ, Schulz AJ, Harris LH, De Wet N, Anderson BA. Abortion attitudes among south Africans: Findings from the 2013 social attitudes survey. Culture, Health & Sexuality. 2017;**19**(8):918-933

[69] Loi UR, Otieno B, Oguttu M, Gemzell Danielsson K, Klingberg-Allvin M, Faxelid E, et al. Abortion and contraceptive use stigma: A cross-sectional study of attitudes and beliefs in secondary school students in western Kenya. Sex Reproductive Health Matters. 2019;**27**(3):1652028

[70] Gelman A, Rosenfeld EA, Nikolajski C, Freedman LR, Steinberg JR, Borrero S. Abortion stigma among abortion-İncome women obtaining abortions in Western Pennsylvania: A qualitative assessment. Perspectives on Sexual and Reproductive Health. 2017;**49**(1):29-36

[71] Esia-Donkoh K, Darteh EKM, Blemano H, Asare H. Who cares? Pre and post abortion experiences among young females in Cape Coast Metropolis, Ghana. African Journal of Reproductive Health. 2015;**19**(2):43-51

[72] Martin LA, Debbink M, Hassinger J, Youatt E, Harris LH. Abortion providers, stigma and professional quality of life. Contraception. 2014;**90**(6):581-587. DOI: 10.1016/j.contraception.2014.07.011

[73] Hulme-Chambers A, Temple-Smith M, Davidson A, Coelli L, Orr C, Tomnay JE. Australian Women's experiences of a rural medical termination of pregnancy service: A qualitative study. Sexual & Reproductive Healthcare. 2018;**15**:23-27

[74] Cockrill K, Biggs A. Can stories reduce abortion stigma? Findings from a longitudinal cohort study. Culture, Health & Sexuality. 2018;**20**(3):335-350. DOI: 10.1080/13691058.2017

[75] Shellenberg KM, Tsui AO. Correlates of perceived and İnternalized stigma among abortion patients in the USA: An exploration by race and Hispanic ethnicity. International Journal of Gynaecology and Obstetrics. 2012;**118**(Suppl. 2):S152-S159

[76] Access to Safe Abortion Critical for Health of Women and Girls. WHO. 2022. Available from: https://www.who.int/news/item/09-03-2022-access-to-safe-abortion-critical-for-health-of-women-and-girls

[77] United Nations World Abortion Policies. United Nations Department of Economic and Social Affairs. New York, NY, March: Population Division; 2011. p. 2011

[78] Center for Reproductive Rights, Abortion Worldwide: Seventeen Years of Reform: Briefing Paper. 2011

[79] Yılmaz B, Şahin N. (2022). Küretaj ve Damgalanma: Bir Sistematik Derleme. Turkiye Klinikleri Journal of Medical Ethics. 2020;**28**(3):451-462. DOI: 10.5336/mdethic.2019-72414

[80] Zordo SD. From Women's 'İrresponsibility' to Foetal 'Patienthood':

Obstetricians-Gynaecologists' perspectives on abortion and İts stigmatisation in Italy and Cataluña. Global Public Health. 2018;**13**(6):711-723

[81] Cárdenas R, Labandera A, Baum SE, Chiribao F, Leus I, Avondet S, et al. "It's something that Marks you": Abortion stigma after decriminalization in Uruguay. Reproductive Health. 2018;**15**(1):150

[82] Aniteye P, O'Brien B, Mayhew SH. Stigmatized by association: Challenges for abortion service providers in Ghana. BMC Health Services Research. 2016;**16**(1):486

[83] Kavanagh A, Wielding S, Cochrane R, Sim J, Johnstone A, Cameron S. 'Abortion' or 'termination of pregnancy'? Views from abortion care providers in Scotland, UK. BMJ Sexual and Reproductive Health. 2018;**44**(2):122-127

[84] Atay H. Kürtaj Yasasının Arkeolojisi: Türkiye'de Kürtaj Düzenlemeleri, Edimleri, Kısıtları ve Mücadele Alanları. Fe Dergi. 2017;**9**:1-16

Section 2

Midwifery Practices

Chapter 2

Midwives' Experience of Traumatic Birth in Cyprus

Eleni Hadjigeorgiou, Ioanna Koliandri and Eva Josephidou

Abstract

In the twenty-first century, research evidence justifies that maternity health professionals, particularly midwives, may experience a birth as traumatic. Childbirth in Cyprus is highly medicalized and midwives as advocates of normal birth, face enormous difficulties to fulfill their professional role. Therefore, identified as crucial to finding more about midwives' experience providing perinatal care in Cyprus. A study was carried out to explore midwives' experiences of traumatic childbirth in Cyprus and how this affects their personal and professional life. Qualitative design approach was used based on Husserl's phenomenological approach. Following ethical approval, data were collected through semi-structured interviews with a purposive sample of midwives (N = 14) from September until December 2021. Data were analyzed using Colaizzi's method and analysis revealed three main themes with subthemes: (1) The nature of traumatic events, (2) Consequences of traumatic experience, and (3) Dealing with traumatic events. Some midwives become defensive and careful, in order to avoid a similar traumatic experience in the future, while some of them develop symptoms of post-traumatic stress disorder (PTSD). Midwives in Cyprus experience traumatic events during childbirth that negatively affect their professional and personal life with long-term effects. Collegiality is important to deal with traumatic events. More awareness must be created during basic and continuing education about decision-making power and problem-solving.

Keywords: midwives, midwifery care, traumatic labor, traumatic birth, perceptions, experiences

1. Introduction

Midwives care for two human beings at the same time and any complication to the mother or the newborn incur uncompensated lesion of the family and community health and prosperity [1]. Midwives providing care during labor and childbirth experience various emotions, such as joy, happiness, and gratitude, sometimes it can lead to sadness and anxiety in the cases midwives are present during traumatic childbirth [2]. The birth process frequently exposes midwives to trauma, which can result in burnout, unmet care, emotional exhaustion, worsening of interpersonal relationships, rise in conflict, dejection, and other problems of a similar nature [3]. A traumatic experience during childbirth can cause stress to health professionals who consequently might develop post-traumatic stress [4]. The symptoms of midwives who have gone through traumatic experiences, however, do not necessarily meet the criteria for PTSD symptoms, even though the concurrent symptoms can have an impact on a person's psychological health [5]. Midwives and pregnant women often develop a special and unique bond, as midwives "coach" pregnant women and support them to have a normal birth and a positive birth experience [4].

There have been numerous research looking into the connection between post-traumatic stress disorder symptoms and midwives' exposure to stressful occurrences during childbirth (PTSD). Sheen et al. [6] conducted research on the relationship between burnout and midwives' exposure to traumatic prenatal events and post-traumatic stress symptoms. From the 421 participants, it was found that the prevalence of PTSD symptoms is at 32% among midwives (n = 138) who reported having experienced a traumatic birth event. Similarly, in Australia, 17% of midwives (n = 102) who witnessed a traumatic birth trauma met criteria for probable PTSD out of the 687 participants [7]. Exposure to a traumatic birth can affect midwives' professional and personal lives but also their mental/psychological health [8].

Previous literature suggests that post-traumatic stress symptoms in midwives have been linked to negative effects on their interactions with women, their ability to care for them, and their ability to make clinical decisions [7]. Halperin et al. [9] identified that midwives often identify traumatic events as a failure, which causes them despair while it can have long-term effects on their mental well-being. It has been found that these events can lead to reduced levels of confidence and an increased tendency to practice defensively [10]. Furthermore, it was identified that the presence of a doctor at a traumatic event could create feelings of degradation in midwives regarding their ability to manage the situation, adding to the stress they experience from the event itself [11]. Innovative strategies are needed to support and assist midwives to cope with traumatic events and at the same time to realize their value and contribution to the care of women [8, 9]. The effects of traumatic occurrences on midwives worldwide include PTSD, compassion fatigue, secondary traumatic stress, and vicarious traumatization [12–15].

In Cyprus, the cesarean section rate is 53.6% in 2018 and 61% in 2022 [16]. Midwives in Cyprus were unable to support and promote physiological birth [17] as they have limited influence on public health policies in relation to the provision of prenatal, intranatal, and postnatal care [18]. Thus, many midwives in Cyprus experience immense stress regarding the medicalization of childbirth, which concludes in facing difficulties in conducting normal childbirth and advocating for women's childbirth rights [17].

The aim of this study was to explore midwives' experiences of traumatic childbirth and how it influenced their personal and professional life.

2. Methodology

Qualitative, descriptive study uses a phenomenological approach according to Husserl's phenomenological approach. The current approach was used because it allows one to gain complete understanding of a topic through truthful reporting and first-hand knowledge. According to Husserl's phenomenological design, the researcher strives for objectivity and to set aside their personal perceptions [19].

2.1 Sample

A purposeful sample of participants was recruited following careful consideration of the need to select midwives; a sample size that would generate quality data. The priority was to achieve depth of data conducive to the production of high-quality findings. The sample consisted of 14 midwives that were recruited from public hospitals and private maternity clinics in Cyprus. The inclusion criteria for participation in the study were: (1) being able to speak and/or understand the Greek language, (2) having at least 5 years' experience in the birth room, (3) being registered as a midwife, and (4) having experienced at least one traumatic birth.

2.2 Ethical issues

Ethical approval was obtained from the Cyprus National Bioethics Committee (ΕΕΒΙΦΕΓΙ/2019/81). All participants completed a consent form containing the assurances for confidentiality, voluntary participation, and their right to withdraw from the study at any stage of the research without any penalty. The participants were assured of their anonymity and privacy while codes were used for each one of them (i.e. Midwife 1, Midwife 2) for data analysis and also for the presentation of the data.

2.3 Data collection

Data collection was achieved through semi-structured one–one interviews with an interview guide developed from relevant literature. The interviews were conducted by one experienced researcher for the consistency of the interviews at a convenient time and place chosen by the participant. A pilot study was carried out with two midwives to evaluate the interview guide in terms of understanding the questions and if they were appropriate. All interviews were face-to-face, where midwives consented with their written permission to participate and for the interviews to be recorded. In addition, it was requested to complete a demographic questionnaire.

2.4 Data analysis

Data analyzed using the Colaizzi method were recognized as the best method for Husserl's phenomenology [20]. Firstly, all the transcribed interviews were read and reread to make sense of them as a whole in order to extract significant statements. The phrases or sentences that directly pertain to the investigated phenomenon were identified. Following is the process of giving meaning to those statements. During this process, pertinent quotes are broadly categorized, where subsequently themes are generated on multiple statements that convey similar meanings. A summarized description of everything generated during the analysis was done so that there is an identification of the fundamental structure of the phenomenon. Lastly, rigor of the data was ensured through discussions with experts and independent reviewers.

2.5 Reflexivity and trustworthiness

A reflective diary was kept by the main researcher during the data collection carefully self-monitoring the impact of biases, beliefs, and personal experiences of the research [21] to ensure rigor and trustworthiness. In addition, COREQ checklist was used to ensure the credibility, trustworthiness, and quality of the study. Data trustworthiness was based on credibility, transferability, dependability, and confirmability. Credibility was established by two authors who had prolonged engagement with the participants and their professional experience. The first author was trained in qualitative methodologies and had 25 years of expertise. To get to an agreement, the authors additionally double-checked and discussed the analysis findings. The interviews were recorded on tape, which increased the dependability of the data by providing a comprehensive and exact account of each participant's responses. Making note of participant quotations to support the findings contributed to ensuring confirmability, which established that themes and categories accurately reflect the participants' experiences and perspectives. Auditability was established by maintaining an audit trail to record the context and background of the study, evaluation of the findings, decisions made, and actions taken during the whole research process.

3. Results

3.1 Demographic findings

In terms of the characteristics of the sample, all 14 participants were permanent residents of the Cyprus Republic working in public hospitals (8) and six private maternity departments. Demographic characteristics of the participants are presented in **Table 1**.

From the in-depth analysis of the data, three themes emerged: (1) The nature of traumatic events, (2) Consequences of traumatic childbirth, and (3) Dealing with traumatic events. Themes and subthemes are shown in **Table 2**.

3.2 The nature of traumatic events

The traumatic events experienced by midwives in the birth room are related to the risk to the mother and the newborn life. The description of the midwives' experiences referred to traumatic events related not only to the mother's life and newborn but also to the medicalization of birth, where complications arose that endangered the life of the mother and the fetus/newborn.

3.2.1 Traumatic events related to mother's life

Midwives' descriptions revealed that when the mother's life was in danger, those events remained vivid in their minds; consequently, having flashbacks and nightmares. The description suggests that these kinds of traumatic events are imprinted in their mind; specifically, a midwife's pain was captured in the case of the loss of a mother.

> *"I cannot forget the death of a woman with amniotic fluid embolism; suddenly she had seizures and after death … we did a cesarean section, but the mother died, and the baby came out alive." (Midwife 3)*

Midwives mentioned that heavy bleeding during labor and birth, was the one of the most traumatic events for them and it was perceived as a traumatizing moment for them.

Characteristics	Number (N = 14)
Place of residence	
Nicosia	10
Larnaca	2
Limassol	1
Famagusta	1
Age	
30–35	4
36–46	2
47–57	4
58–65	4
Marital status	
Married	12
In a relationship	2
Education	
Postgraduate	6
Masters	6
Doctoral students	2
Years of experience	
>20 years	4
11–20 years	6
5–10 years	4

Table 1.
Socio-demographic characteristics of participants.

> *" ..mother has a massive bleeding … ., I had never seen such hemorrhage in the many years I have been working." (Midwife 4)*

> *"An uncontrollable bleeding had started, where … . it was very shocking (embarrassing smile), I had never seen so much blood … the woman was in the operating room and the blood dropped … on the floor." (Midwife 6)*

3.2.2 Traumatic events related to newborn's health

Some midwives reported traumatic events related to the newborn's health complications and/or death. One midwife had described the agony she had experienced, to keep the newborn alive, but the newborn passed away the next day.

> *"The baby was born alive but in bad condition … the next day he/she died. I felt guilty, I blamed myself." (Midwife 7)*

Similarly, another midwife reported the death of the newborn that was imprinted in their mind and explained that it was due to severe and sudden bleeding.

Themes	Subthemes
1. The nature of traumatic events	1.1 Related to mothers' health
	1.2 Related to newborn's health
	1.3 Related to medicalization of birth
2.Consequences of traumatic experience	2.1 Short-term psychological effects 2.2 Long-term psychological effects
	2.3 Implications on the professional life
3. Dealing with traumatic events	3.1 Colleague support and/or family support in dealing with traumatic events
	3.2 Personal characteristics

Table 2.
Themes and subthemes of the findings.

> *"I cannot forget the death of a baby; the mother came to the hospital with a sudden hemorrhage, we could not save the baby." (Midwife 11)*

3.2.3 Traumatic events related to medicalization of birth

Midwives strongly pointed out the fact that in some cases during labor and birth, they did not offer evidence-based care to the mother as they were afraid to create conflict with the obstetrician. A midwife gave a vivid description of a disagreement with the obstetrician as he wished to expedite the birth and made interventions to speed up the birth.

> *"Obstetrician told me that he will make a "milkshake of drugs", I will put that in the woman's vein and by the end the cervix will be dilated very easily, and birth will finish easily... it was a traumatic experience because I was next to the woman ...and by the end she had Vacuum extraction." (Midwife 13)*

Vacuum extraction was also described by some midwives as a traumatic experience for mothers' and babies' health. Specifically, they explained a certain event where the suction cup of the vacuum extraction was used several times does not feed well and does not facilitate the birth of the baby.

> *"The doctor tried several times to apply the suction cup on the baby head and pull it out; we tried to stop him, but he would not hear. The poor woman was screaming in pain..." (Midwife 12)*

In addition, midwives mentioned that some obstetricians' behavior in their opinion was unprofessional. A certain event was described by a midwife in which she was present where misconduct took place. The authority of the obstetrician was imposed rather than the midwife's opinion and mother's wishes.

> *"He put her to bed, the woman cried from the pain, she was telling him: I'm in pain do not touch me and he continues and asks her to push ..." (Midwife 13)*

> *"The woman said to us that she wishes to have no intervention during labor, no oxytocin, no epidural but the obstetrician convinced her to start Oxytocin and have*

> *an epidural. I could not react; I stay speechless but then I felt so disappointed with herself." (Midwife 7)*

3.3 Consequences of traumatic childbirth

3.3.1 Short-term psychological effects

The most prominent effect of being present at a traumatic birth was psychological, through the traumatic experience, midwives had short-term psychological effects. Many of the symptoms were related to PTSD symptoms but none of them were diagnosed with PTSD by a professional. Specifically, it was reported that they felt "numb," a state of constant vigilance to surroundings (hyperarousal), had negative beliefs about themselves, had dark moods, felt very nervous, had tachycardia, and were frustrated. Some midwives felt very bad because they did not react to situations that caused trauma to women or new-born and they remained speechless. Some of the midwives reported being present at events where obstetric violence took place and subsequently their stress increased.

> *"I felt a lot of remorse, I did not want to talk about it, I did not want to listen, I did not want to talk about it, I did not sleep at night, I felt very bad, because if I felt that I could not do what I want to help that baby." (Midwife 8)*

> *"Most of the time I find myself coming home, with stress, I reflect on the event to see what went wrong... I recognise obstetric violence and that causes me more stress." (Midwife 2)*

Midwives develop somatic symptoms such as tachycardia, headaches, and sleep disturbances/nightmares and felt very bad and guilty as they did not protect women, which affected their morale and made them feel weak, sad, and fearful.

> *"I was praying, I felt bad as I was discussing the incident with my husband." (Midwife 11)*

> *"I felt bad, I felt guilty, I could not protect the woman." (Midwife 12)*

> *"A lady admitted with placenta praevia. We took her to the theater for cesarean section, we saved the mother but not the baby. I could not forget that scene and after that, I had sleep disturbances." (Midwife 8)*

> *"The baby was born but I had a headache and slowly - slowly, now I have tachycardia." (Midwife 4)*

3.3.2 Long-term psychological effects

Long-term effects of traumatic events such as flashbacks, depression, low esteem, and thoughts of leaving the birth department to be away from childbirth were reported by midwives. Midwives were stressed out and reported not feeling well for years, while others mentioned experiencing depressive symptoms.

> *"For years ... I felt very bad... I think I was in the early stages of depression. I always had that incident in my mind." (Midwife 4)*

> *"I work for many years in the birthing room but after traumatic events, I feel so stressed that make me feel sick." (Midwife 7)*

> *"That scene of women crying in pain after vacuum extraction, stay in my mind and made me feel so miserable, I found myself to prefer to stay at home doing nothing. , I cannot describe my feelings." (Midwife 10)*

Furthermore, two midwives could not forget traumatic events that occurred when they were students, doing their internship in the hospital. They felt that as students they could not react, but this experience remained in their minds. Specifically, they stated that they had nightmares.

> *"I had bad dreams; I remember everything very well and that affected my professional life." (Midwife 13)*

> *"I was in the birth room and the woman was fully dilated and the obstetrician shouted to her to push and push... and one of my colleagues - a midwife went next to her pushed her uterus without informing her and said "I help you I help you" . After that I had nightmares ..." (Midwife 7)*

> *"After I saw the baby come out after cesarean section dead, I felt so bad that I could not sleep. I had nightmares." (Midwife 4)*

3.3.3 Implications on professional life

The implications for professional life were many. Descriptions suggest that midwives blame themselves, they feel guilty and have constant fear of future errors and feelings of inadequacy, loss of confidence and entering a vicious cycle with increased odds of future self-perceived errors, have been shown to be consequences of being involved in a severe event and the event lowered their self-esteem, their care. Some of them wanted to take sick leave and be away from their work while others mentioned that they changed their place of work and prefer to work in a nursery. Some midwives reported that they felt alone, while they had experienced a traumatic event, they were afraid to discuss the whole event with their colleagues because they were afraid of the criticism. Specifically, one midwife mentioned that she was present in a difficult birth and that neonate suffered a lot and she went home and continuously had this event in their mind.

> *"I went home and I have in my mind the whole event continuously, the poor baby suffers .. I have it now in front of my eyes ... the ventouse." (Midwife 7)*

Some midwives opined that there are changes in maternity care and in the passing years their role and work culture were affected negatively. Midwives' autonomous role to create special relationships with women and advocate for their childbirth rights got lost. Obstetricians wish to be present during normal childbirth and if everything went well, they get all the credit from the system, from the relatives, and the contribution of the midwife. But at the same time if something goes wrong, then they blame the midwife. In this way, midwives are forced to change their clinical practice so that they are in line with the mindset of doctors.

> *"Sometimes during labor and birth, there is a very high level of stress ..... if something goes well during the birth, okay, all credits went to the doctor, if something goes wrong, it is the midwife's fault ..." (Midwife 2)*

Some descriptions reflected the work environment where midwives felt that there was no adequate coordination or support and not working as a team, which often led to missed care.

> *"The work culture where we as midwives worked more as a team no longer exists ..... There is a lack of coordination, due to bad management. we have no leaders."(Midwife 14)*

In contrast, some midwives emphasized that the support they receive from other midwives helps them to feel better.

3.4 Dealing with traumatic events

3.4.1 Colleague support and/or family support in dealing with traumatic events

Support in dealing with traumatic events came either from their colleagues and/or their family. After the event, some of the midwives shared with their colleagues their feelings, thoughts, and concerns and discussed with them the event and their reactions.

> *"I had support from other midwives, listened to me because .. listening is a kind of support, then they advised me ... they helped me a lot just talking ...." (Midwife 13)*

Midwives reported that after experiencing a traumatic event they found family support beneficial. Midwives refer to their spouse or partner support.

> *"I discussed the event with my husband ..he helped me." (Midwife 11)*

3.4.2 Personal characteristics

Midwives react to traumatic events in many ways according to their personalities and they refer to personal characteristics that helped them deal with traumatic events. An experienced midwife based on her expertise.

> *"When I saw a lot of blood on the bed I said to myself you know what to do and you must do it ... , think, concentrate on your knowledge ..." (Midwife 1)*

Midwives became stronger and learned how to react to similar events, pay attention to the smallest details, acted more autonomously, and became more accountable.

> *"Traumatic events help me to pay more attention to some details during midwifery care. I will improve my skills to be able to cope with something similar in the future ..." (Midwife 5)*

> *"That event gives me strength... If I have to deal with the same situation again, I will try to think better, a strength comes inside me now." (Midwife 2)*

4. Discussion

This study explored midwives' experiences of traumatic birth while identifying the implications on their personal and professional life. Midwives had described the various traumatic events they experienced, which entailed exposure to emotionally demanding situations, how their lives were affected, describing their reactions and feelings. Cope mechanism with a traumatic event developed, while some midwives mentioned that nothing could help them and had partially changed their place of work and clinical practice. A traumatic perinatal event was defined as occurring during labor or shortly after birth when the midwife perceived the mother or her infant to be at risk and they (the midwife) had experienced fear, helplessness, or horror in response [22].

PTSD is characterized by involuntary and distressing recollections of the traumatic event (e.g., flashbacks and intrusive imagery), avoidance of reminders (people, places, and thoughts) of the event, heightened arousal (where concentration and sleep can be disrupted), and alterations to worldview beliefs and affective states (e.g., guilt, fear, or shame). The psychological effects on midwives are important for their mental health. Midwives exposed to a traumatic birth develop symptoms of post-traumatic Stress disorder (PTSD) [23, 24]. PTSD did not emerge in our interviews but high levels of stress and in one case symptoms of depression were prevalent in the midwives. Halperin et al. [9] reported the long-term effects of traumatic births on midwives where they dealt with guilt and nightmares regarding the traumatic event, which was consistent with the findings of our study. The fear, stress, and guilt led women to believe that the traumatic events women experienced were their fault [22].

The effects of abusive care were discussed in detail by midwives, including bodily integrity violations, unnecessary roughness, witnessing or participating in procedures that were not in the woman's or the baby's best interests, and general interpersonal disrespect in which the woman's dignity was disregarded or her wishes were ignored [25]. This also consisted in the current study, descriptions of abusive care and the authority figures that affected the midwives. Cankaya et al. [26] identified that midwives tried to be more defensive and careful, so they would avoid a similar traumatic experience in the future. Also, it was pointed out that, sometimes due to management, coordination and communications problems occurred, where most of the time obstetricians had no consequences for their actions. As a result, midwives changed their care, and they did not react if interventions occurred during childbirth. Traumatic events were associated with emotional distress in midwives, specifically, feelings of worry, guilt, anger, and horror regarding the event the pregnant women experienced under their care [7].

It has been observed that long-term effects on midwives' personal lives are consistent with other studies; some of the midwives reported experiencing feelings of guilt and having nightmares about the traumatic event they experience while others tried to avoid any situations that would put them in the same position [9, 27]. In certain cases, there were immediate effects that affected their personal life such as stress, fear, and sadness because they felt responsible for the event [22].

The support from their co-workers, family, and friends was of important value for the midwives and had a vital role in adapting resilience in the workplace.

Another factor effective in resilience was the sense of usefulness and reassurance. Halperin's study [9] justified that emotional support by coworkers and family were essential for their emotional well-being, to cope with the traumatic event but also in reaffirming their professionalism. Specifically, family support was the most important support system [26]. In contrast, in some cases, the events were criticized by their coworkers, which made it more difficult for them to process [28].

Furthermore, another factor that contributed to dealing with the traumatic experiences was the additional information given, as well as the education of the midwives, on issues that they felt had gaps. This factor was shown through the study of Wahlberg et al. [2] that it is important since midwives need training to increase their resilience on an individual and professional level. It is important to have multidisciplinary professional meetings, in which midwives can discuss their traumatic experiences and have therapeutic discussions with them. Professional support should be provided to midwives to deal with traumatic experiences, recognize and understand the impact of psychological trauma, and have the appropriate support to provide quality perinatal care [26].

5. Conclusion

Midwives living in Cyprus experience many traumatic events, significant ones being bleeding before or after childbirth, death of the mother, and the death of the newborn and unnecessary interventions. It has also become evident that vacuum extraction and the medicalization of childbirth and lack of support affect the mental health of midwives. Midwives following the experience of a traumatic perinatal event need effective support at both a personal and organizational level.

Regarding the effects of midwives after the traumatic experiences, they had a significant impact on both their personal and professional lives. They pointed out that the short psychological effects they had were related to the fear they felt after the traumatic event, and they considered themselves responsible for it. Long-term effects were reported such as symptoms of depression and high levels of stress and PTSD, which was distressing to the midwives. The study showed that midwives, experiencing a traumatic experience in the birth room, forced themselves to change their place of work and clinical practice. Factors that contributed positively to coping with these events were the mutual support from other midwives and their families.

The consequences of traumatic births on midwives affect their professional and personal life. It should be feasible to seek professional help when experiencing these kinds of events to share their worries and experiences with suitable care and therapy. Educational programs and seminars are needed not only to educate midwives but also to empower them to help improve the outcomes of traumatic events. Most importantly, multidisciplinary intervention groups should be implemented where midwives could share their experiences and discuss their worries with other coworkers to help them recognize that they are not alone. It is vital for the health systems to provide counseling or multidisciplinary meetings where they can discuss responses to trauma in a nonjudgmental way and provide them with information on how to access support if desired or needed. Conclusively, there is an urgent need to facilitate development of health professionals that feel confident and competent in providing the right evidence-based perinatal care.

Acknowledgements

I acknowledge the generosity of midwives in Cyprus for their time and willingness to share with us their experiences from a traumatic birth.

Conflict of interest

The authors declare no conflict of interest.

Notes/thanks/other declarations

Special thanks to all the midwives who participated and offered valuable data. Warm thanks to MSc students for their significant contribution to identifying the problems that midwives experience.

Author details

Eleni Hadjigeorgiou*, Ioanna Koliandri and Eva Josephidou
Department of Nursing, School of Health Sciences, Cyprus University of Technology, Limassol, Cyprus

*Address all correspondence to: eleni.hadjigeorgiou@cut.ac.cy

References

[1] Leinweber J, Rowe HJ. The costs of 'being with the woman': Secondary traumatic stress in midwifery. Midwifery. 2010;**26**(1):76-87

[2] Wahlberg Å, Andreen Sachs M, Johannesson K, Hallberg G, Jonsson M, Skoog Svanberg A, et al. Post-traumatic stress symptoms in Swedish obstetricians and midwives after severe obstetric events: A cross-sectional retrospective survey. BJOG: An International Journal of Obstetrics & Gynaecology. 2017;**124**(8):1264-1271

[3] Martínez-Serrano P, Palmar-Santos AM, Solís-Muñoz M, Álvarez-Plaza C, Pedraz-Marcos A. Midwives' experience of delivery care in late foetal death: A qualitative study. Midwifery. 2018;**66**:127-133

[4] von Schantz-Enoksson H. Midwives Ways of Coping with Crises [Master Thesis]. 2018. Available from: https://www.theseus.fi/bitstream/handle/10024/143819/vonSchantz-Enoksson_Henrika.pdf?sequence=1

[5] Fontein-Kuipers Y, Duivis H, Schamper V, Schmitz V, Stam A, Koster D. Reports of work-related traumatic events: A mixed methods study. European Journal of Midwifery. 2018;**2**(18):1-9

[6] Sheen K, Spiby H, Slade P. Exposure to traumatic perinatal experiences and post-traumatic stress symptoms in midwives: prevalence and association with burnout. International Journal of Nursing Studies. 2015;**52**(2):578-587

[7] Leinweber J, Creedy DK, Rowe H, Gamble J. Responses to birth trauma and prevalence of post-traumatic stress among Australian midwives. Women and Birth. 2017;**30**(1):40-45

[8] Slade P, West H, Thomson G, Lane S, Spiby H, Edwards RT, et al. STRAWB2 (Stress and Wellbeing After Childbirth): A randomised controlled trial of targeted self-help materials to prevent post-traumatic stress disorder following childbirth. BJOG: An International Journal of Obstetrics & Gynaecology. 2020;**127**(7):886-896

[9] Halperin O, Goldblatt H, Noble A, Raz I, Zvulunov I, Liebergall WM. Stressful childbirth situations: A qualitative study of midwives. Journal of Midwifery & Women's Health. 2011;**56**(4):388-394

[10] Elmir R, Pangas J, Dahlen H, Schmied V. A meta-ethnographic synthesis of midwives' and nurses' experiences of adverse labour and birth events. Journal of Clinical Nursing. 2017;**26**(23-24):4184-4200

[11] Aydın R, Aktaş S. Midwives' experiences of traumatic births: A systematic review and meta-synthesis. European Journal of Midwifery. 2021;**5**:1-10

[12] Sabo BM. Compassion fatigue and nursing work: Can we accurately capture the consequences of caring work? International Journal of Nursing Practice. 2006;**12**(3):136-142

[13] Devilly GJ, Wright R, Varker T. Vicarious trauma, secondary traumatic stress or simply burnout? Effect of trauma therapy on mental health professionals. Australian & New Zealand Journal of Psychiatry. 2009;**43**(4):373-385

[14] Newell JM, MacNeil GA. Professional burnout, vicarious trauma, secondary traumatic stress, and compassion

fatigue. Best Practices in Mental Health. 2010;**6**(2):57-68

[15] Showalter SE. Compassion fatigue: What is it? Why does it matter? Recognizing the symptoms, acknowledging the impact, developing the tools to prevent compassion fatigue, and strengthen the professional already suffering from the effects. American Journal of Hospice and Palliative Medicine®. 2010;**27**(4):239-242

[16] Ministry of Health. Republic of Cyprus. Cyprus public and private maternity units. Important perinatal health indicators for the year 2014-2018. Health Monitoring Unit. 2018:1-36. Available from: https://www.moh.gov.cy/Moh/MOH.nsf/All/1A26898D0CD56210C22579C600278E4B/$file/Perinatal%20health%20in%20Cyprus_Important%20Indicators%202014-2018.pdf

[17] Hadjigeorgiou E, Spyridou A, Christoforou A, Iannuzzi L, Giovinale S, Canepa MM, et al. Variation in caes are an section rates in Cyprus, Italy and Iceland: An analysis of the role of the media. Minerva Ginecologica. 2018;**70**(6):676-686

[18] Hadjigeorgiou E, Christofi MD. How midwifery education in Cyprus has evolved in response to the demands of a complex and changing world. The Practicing Midwife. 2018;**21**(8):39-42

[19] Gutland C. Husserlian phenomenology as a kind of introspection. Frontiers in Psychology. 2018;**9**:896

[20] Colaizzi PF. Psychological Research as the Phenomenologist Views it. In: Valle RS, King M, editors. Existential-Phenomenological Alternatives for Psychology. Oxford University Press; 1978. p. 6

[21] Berger R. Now I see it, now I don't: Researcher's position and reflexivity in qualitative research. Qualitative Research. 2015;**15**(2):219-234

[22] Sheen K, Spiby H, Slade P. What are the characteristics of perinatal events perceived to be traumatic by midwives? Midwifery. 2016;**40**:55-61

[23] Toohill J, Fenwick J, Sidebotham M, Gamble J, Creedy DK. Trauma and fear in Australian midwives. Women and Birth. 2019;**32**(1):64-71

[24] Cohen R, Leykin D, Golan-Hadari D, Lahad M. Exposure to traumatic events at work, posttraumatic symptoms and professional quality of life among midwives. Midwifery. 2017;**50**:1-8

[25] Arksey H, O'Malley L. Scoping studies: Towards a methodological framework. International Journal of Social Research Methodology. 2005;**8**(1):19-32

[26] Cankaya S, Erkal Aksoy Y, Dereli YS. Midwives' experiences of witnessing traumatic hospital birth events: A qualitative study. Journal of Evaluation in Clinical Practice. 2021;**27**(4):847-857

[27] Minooee S, Cummins A, Foureur M, Travaglia J. Catastrophic thinking: Is it the legacy of traumatic births? Midwives' experiences of shoulder dystocia complicated births. Women and Birth. 2021;**34**(1):e38-e46

[28] Javid N, Ahmadi A, Mirzaei M, Atghaei M. Effectiveness of solution-focused group counseling on the mental health of midwifery students. Revista Brasileira de Ginecologia e Obstetrícia. 2019;**41**:500-507

Chapter 3

Dynamics of the Twenty-First-Century Midwifery Practice

Jackline Ayikoru, Akello Harriet, Raymond Otim and Pebolo Francis Pebalo

Abstract

Globally, midwifery is the safest, most cost-effective, and most satisfying method of birth assistance. This age-old profession embraces the most non-interventionist philosophy that childbirth is a natural and normal process in which the attendant merely assists in the healthy routine progression. Midwifery is commonly assumed to be all about assisting labor and childbirth, but there is more to it than that. This noble profession entails skilled, knowledgeable, and compassionate care for childbearing women, newborn infants, and families across the continuum throughout pre-pregnancy, and pre, intra, and postpartum periods. Over decades, midwifery has evolved from being informal and invisible to independent professional practice with major shifts in the scope of practice, gender, economic, and career dynamics concerning the profession. With maternal and child health being at the center of most important developments, the midwife stands out in his/her role as a primary care provider, advocate, and teacher.

Keywords: midwifery, midwife, current trends, practice, roles, technology

1. Introduction

The practice of midwifery worldwide is the safest, most cost-effective, and most satisfying method of birth assistance. This age-old profession embraces the most non-interventionist philosophy that childbirth is a natural and normal process in which the attendant merely assists in the healthy routine progression [1].

Midwifery is commonly assumed to be all about assisting labor and childbirth, but there is more to it than that. This noble profession entails skilled, knowledgeable, and compassionate care for childbearing women, newborn infants, and families across the continuum throughout pre-pregnancy, pregnancy, birth, postpartum, and the early weeks of life. Additionally, the scope of midwifery practice includes family planning and the provision of reproductive health services. Midwifery services are a core part of universal health coverage, not a narrow segment. These services extend beyond the confines of the hospital settings to the communities and beyond [2]. This ancient art has evolved over centuries from being an informal practice to being an advanced, globally recognized, and regulated professional practice in the twenty-first century [3]. This chapter presents highlights of midwifery and key advances in the profession in this age.

2. History of midwifery

One of the most ancient fields of art, the origin of midwifery dates back to the ancient stone age era around 40,000 Before Christ (BC), through the dark ages, the Biblical era, up to date. Women have always instinctively supported each other during pregnancy and childbirth [4]. In the Paleolithic age (50,000–9000 BC), women supported each other during childbirth based on observation of behaviors of animals such as squatting while giving birth, cutting the umbilical cord to separate the mother from the newborn, providing warmth to the infant, and initiating breastfeeding [5]. The Biblical era also termed the golden era between 2200 BC–1700 BC upheld midwifery as a socially respectable art practiced by women who managed normal pregnancies and deliveries by performing skilled vaginal examinations, with religion and witchcraft as a basis of practice brought forth women's empowerment, family-centered care, and key milestones in the development of professionalism in midwifery practice [5, 6]. Midwifery in the modern era (seventeenth to eighteenth century) saw major advances like instrumental deliveries for difficult births and training of males in midwife-training institutions [7, 8]. Throughout the nineteenth century before the evolution of the nursing profession, midwives remained the main provider of obstetric care services in most countries [9]. From the twentieth to the current twenty-first-century change has been a constant occurrence in all arenas of human development including cultures, societies, technologies, and knowledge and this is reciprocated in the evolution of midwifery too [10].

3. The role of a midwife

Over decades, midwifery has evolved from being informal and invisible to independent professional practice with major shifts in the scope of practice, gender, economic, and career dynamics concerning the profession. New and expanded roles in midwifery practice are key to the provision of high-quality care and professionalism [11]. Maternal and child health being at the center of most important developments, the midwife stands out in his/her role as a primary care provider, advocate, and teacher as they provide multidisciplinary, non-hierarchical patient-centered care to their clients [12].

Health promotion is one of the key roles played by a midwife [13] some of which include Health education, screening, immunization, prophylactic treatments, contraception, and domiciliary care services. Midwives are taking a leading role in developing, implementing, and evaluating these new models of care to ensure that they reflect the principles of women-centered continuity of midwifery care. At the policy level, midwives are also influencing changes in systems of care and service birth [14].

4. Current trends in midwifery

4.1 Regulation of practice

As a matter of course, midwifery was an unregulated art that involved females taking initiatives informed by their society's needs and previous practices passed on from elderly women [9]. These traditional birth attendants(midwives) have been an integral part of pregnancy and childbirth to this day and some parts of the globe have taken the initiative to provide basic formal training to them. This integrates them into the healthcare system and encourages collaboration, allowing them to be able to identify abnormalities and provide early referrals to qualified professionals. Being a predominantly female profession, midwives struggled to achieve due recognition given the status of women in society at that time. This backdrop and fear of extinction of the practice gave birth to a movement that later on came to be known as the International Midwives Union (IMU) [4, 9].

The international confederation of Midwives (ICM) which was formed from the International Midwives' Union (IMU) in 1922 is an international umbrella that unites midwives and midwifery organizations in various countries across all the continents across the globe. In 2011, the International Confederation of Midwives released Global Standards for Midwifery Education, Regulation, and Association, guiding international midwifery for the first time [15]. However specific regulation of the profession, the scope of practice, and training are variable in the different countries worldwide [4].

Regulation of midwifery practice varies from place to place. In the African continent, Stakeholders such as nursing associations and academicians have varied and complementary roles concerning reforming professional practice and education regulation [16]. Nursing and Midwifery Council (NMC) has powers to regulate midwifery and nursing in the United Kingdom. The council retains the powers to establish and maintain a register of all qualified midwives, and to take needed action in case set standards are questioned [17]. In Australia, the recognition of midwifery as a separate profession from nursing has been a recent phenomenon and has been surrounded by considerable debate and discussion within both professions [14]. Today, midwifery gallantly stands out as a profession that has a regulated scope of practice [18] with well-organized and recognized structures.

4.2 Gender dynamics

The word woman from which "midwife" is coined is frequently associated with care and empathy while "man" is more often associated with masculine roles such as protection and provision, so originally only women were involved in childbirth and all that was entailed in caring for a pregnant woman. However, that has changed in our era, Key advances in the practice include male involvement (men-wifery), which was unheard of in a predominantly female profession. More males than ever have ventured into and embraced midwifery as a career.

This transition has been faced with criticism and fears from women, husbands, communities, regulatory bodies, policymakers, and even the health workforce to date.

Even as much as males have ventured into the profession, we cannot conclude that there is diversity. In the United States, only 2% of midwives are male [19] while in Afghanistan, Brunei, Cambodia, Japan, and Saudi Arabia males are completely prohibited from enrolling for midwifery for cultural and religious reasons [20]. In the Ugandan context, male midwives are only trained from bachelorette level and beyond, certificate and diploma training is open to nursing and other professions, except midwifery [21].

4.3 Scope of practice

Being one of the most diverse professions of all time, there is a medley of roles encompassed in midwifery today; from being birth assistants (clinical practice) primarily to comprehensive maternal and child care. The triad of competition from doctors (obstetricians/gynecologists), increased hospital deliveries, and advancements in medical interventions such as cesarean section, labor monitoring, vacuum assisted delivery have rather reshaped the practice of a midwife [9]. The midwife is now not only concerned with providing direct clinical care during pregnancy and childbirth but even her family and community she hails from, provision of other sexual and reproductive health services, research, academia, leadership, policy formation, and even more roles.

4.4 Technology in healthcare

While the rest of the world enjoys advances in technological development, reproductive health is not spared. Assisted Reproductive Technologies (ART) have sprouted in various forms to make it easier for infertile women to enjoy the privilege of parenthood, complex diagnostic procedures, advanced treatment and monitoring options, and beyond.

Invitro fertilization, genetic engineering, cloning, surrogacy, artificial wombs, and various other modifications in the modes of reproduction have birthed major shifts in the type and mode of care provided to clients, as well as a range of ethical issues that the midwife must negotiate in the daily practice of the profession. While ARTs have become more normalized as a means of achieving parenthood, there may be associated risks. Midwives, as the main caregivers for pregnant women need to be well informed, and mindful of the potential risks to the mother and her baby whilst providing care that is the most appropriate and supportive, to enable these women to achieve a safe and satisfying childbirth experience [22].

4.5 Ethical issues arising

The Hippocratic oath forms an ethical foundation that governs morally acceptable midwifery practice through principles such as respect for persons, justice, beneficence, and non-maleficence which often conflict with the morals of individual professionals, patients, health system policies, cultural and societal norms, and several other factors and result in ethical dilemmas [23, 24]. Such include issues surrounding informed consent, surrogacy, shared decision making, patient preference vis a vis professional recommendation, religious and cultural conflicts with professional care.

Therefore, continuous increases in the level of education coupled with technological advances present a need to improve and updated professional and ethical codes that guide conduct and professional practice [25].

4.6 Midwife-led care

The term mid-wife-led care is a model of patient care where a midwife is the lead health-professional responsible for the planning, organization, and delivery of care given to a woman and her family during preconception, antenatal care, delivery, and through the postnatal period. It ensures woman-centered care and advocates for minimal interventions on assumptions that pregnancy and childbirth are normal events [26, 27]. This model is based on the perception that pregnancy and childbirth are naturally occurring physiological processes and it is associated with better client outcomes, high effectiveness, and efficiency among professionals [28–30].

However, due to socio-cultural factors, overlap in professional roles and responsibilities among various health professionals [31], and medicalization of childbirth and reproductive health services midwives are placed in a passive role in regards to the scope of work they should making it challenging to fully achieve midwife-led care [28].

4.7 Advances in education, research, and advocacy

Nursing and midwifery form the backbone of health service delivery and patient satisfaction depending on their competencies [32]. They can help countries optimally contribute to achieving universal health coverage, equity, and other population health goals. This section's emphasis however is on the midwife - their training, research, and advocacy relevance regarding their practice.

4.8 Education

There are various levels of midwifery training, and what distinguishes them is the quality of practice each does in a role [33]. Here is a list of levels and their differences.

Level 1: Basic Midwifery- The midwife performs elementary midwifery skills but cannot perform any other additional skills beyond what is required for conducting normal deliveries.

Level 2: Advanced Midwifery- A midwife provides basic skills to deliver the baby and can also perform other basic medical care besides delivery.

Level 3: Advanced Midwifery with Advanced Practice- Midwife provides skills to deliver the baby including difficult deliveries perform medical care and do advanced midwifery skills which may involve research, advocacy, and public health.

Level 4: Advanced Midwifery with Advanced Practice and Advanced Service Delivery- the midwife provides skills to deliver a baby including all difficult deliveries performs advanced midwifery skills including research, advocacy, public health, and education, and demonstrates advanced service delivery models.

Of note, the best midwives are not necessarily the ones with the most training highest level of certification. A good midwife rather pays attention to the detail of the person in front of them. They listen to their concerns, take care of their needs and do everything they can to make the time they spend with them as comfortable as possible. A qualified midwife is skilled in the care of a woman and their babies at/during childbirth and can provide medical care and comfort to a woman during childbirth. Today midwives are qualified by having a higher education certification, diploma, or degree, however, qualification is not only about being able to pass exams but explicit exhibition of quality care and or service delivery.

4.9 What is happening?

The midwifery profession is evolving despite various qualifications and cadres of midwifery training- and what differentiates them is the quality of output each does on a role. When you go through these roles, it's not just a matter of how long you have been studying but - *how much you have learned, how well you have been trained, and how much you have had to work for it*.

Right now, the midwifery profession is going through a transition trying to recognize the value of work that is being done by valuing the knowledge and skills being passed on. We are taking what has been traditionally seen as a profession and making it into a more - *respected and valued profession.*

4.10 Research

Being a focal point of maternal care, midwives ought to continuously strive towards providing individualized, appropriate, family-centered care, prioritizing not only the women but also their families, communities, and social and cultural backgrounds. If care is to be appropriate and effective, there needs to be an assessment at a community and individual level, this is what makes practice and service delivery advanced and different – being able to realize patient needs beyond physical conditions and advocate for patient needs through root cause analysis. Health needs assessment is a systematic method for reviewing the health issues facing a population, which informs policy and sets priorities for appropriate resources to improve health and reduce inequalities [34].

4.11 To achieve this - advocacy

You will need the information to persuade policymakers to change their policies, laws, or implementation, whether through direct lobbying or other means such as provoking an official investigation or influencing public opinion [35]. You will need to conduct somewhat research to obtain this preliminary survey information. This in turn requires advanced research skills and expressiveness in communication when caring for the patient and her relatives.

To be concise, this presents an opportunity to engage with local communities, other healthcare providers, and commissioners, and provides the evidence to plan appropriate services, targeted at those most in need - improving health service delivery and health equity in such needy communities.

The section sought to stress the importance of education, research, and advocacy concerning the midwifery practice in addressing the key health challenges today by equipping the midwife with the necessary tools to promote health equity.

4.12 Gap - research

Currently, there is a scarcity of research in midwifery practice which if not dealt with promptly may result in a disastrous glitch after a given period vis-à-vis the expected roles of the midwife firstly in clinical practice, research, and advocacy in promoting evidence-based quality care to patients to achieve health equity and universal health coverage [36].

It is important therefore to note that, research and innovation remain the basic cornerstone upon which new advancements and guidelines for clinical practice are based and developed [37]. The provision of adequate health care for the finest patient management outcomes is pivoted on the interplay between unwavering clinical practice and medical research without ignoring advocacy for marginalized people to promote health equity in care and practice.

5. Conclusion

"In all cultures, the midwife's place is on the threshold of life, where intense emotions, fear, hope, longing, triumph, and incredible physical power enable a new human being to emerge. Her vocation is unique"- Sheila Kitzinger.

Therefore, as man lives in a changing society so does his environment, culture, and practices in reciprocity. Midwifery, being one of the most ancient professions has experienced revolutionization over the ages as knowledge advances, cultures, and societies and this has led to a more organized and recognized global profession, but its goal remains to promote the well-being of the woman and her baby.

Author details

Jackline Ayikoru[1*], Akello Harriet[2], Raymond Otim[1] and Pebolo Francis Pebalo[1]

1 Gulu University, Gulu, Uganda

2 St. Mary's Hospital Lacor, Gulu, Uganda

*Address all correspondence to: ayikoruhopejackline@gmail.com

References

[1] Rifkin D. Midwifery: An international perspective--the need for universal legal recognition. Indiana Journal of Global Legal Studies. 1997;**4**:509-536

[2] Horton R, Astudillo O. The power of midwifery. Lancet. 2014;**384**(9948):1075-1076

[3] Hammick M, et al. Being Interprofessional. Polity. 2009

[4] ICM. The Origins of Midwifery. 2018.

[5] Towler J, Bramall J. Midwives in History and Society. London: Taylor & Francis; 2023

[6] Barnawi N, Richter S, Habib F. Midwifery and midwives: A historical analysis. Journal of Research in Nursing and Midwifery. 2013;**2**(8):114-121

[7] Stern C. MIDWIVES, MALE-MIDWIVES, AND NURSE-MIDWIVES: An epitome of relationships and roles. Obstetrics & Gynecology. 1972;**39**(2):308-322

[8] Kontoyannis M, Katsetos C. Midwives in early modern Europe (1400-1800). Health Science Journal. 2011;**5**(1):31

[9] Marland H, Rafferty AM. Midwives, Society and Childbirth: Debates and Controversies in the Modern Period. London: Routledge; 2002

[10] Leap N, Hunter B. The midwife's Tale: An Oral History from Handywoman to Professional Midwife. South Yorkshire: Pen and Sword; 2013

[11] Goemaes R et al. Advanced midwifery practice: An evolutionary concept analysis. Midwifery. 2016;**42**:29-37

[12] Walsh D, Steen M. The role of the midwife: Time for a review: Reader in midwifery Denis Walsh and research fellow in midwifery Mary Steen at the University of Central Lancashire and the RCM examine both the current situation of impersonalised midwifery and the ideal of combining holistic care with evidence-based practice. Midwives Magazine. 2007;**10**(7):320-324

[13] Beldon A, Crozier S. Health promotion in pregnancy: The role of the midwife. The Journal of the Royal Society for the Promotion of Health. 2005;**125**(5):216-220

[14] Homer CS et al. The role of the midwife in Australia: Views of women and midwives. Midwifery. 2009;**25**(6):673-681

[15] Kennedy HP et al. United States model midwifery legislation and regulation: Development of a consensus document. Journal of Midwifery & Women's Health. 2018;**63**(6):652-659

[16] McCarthy CF et al. Nursing and midwifery regulatory reform in east, central, and southern Africa: A survey of key stakeholders. Human Resources for Health. 2013;**11**(1):1-7

[17] Baird B et al. Midwifery Regulation in the United Kingdom. London, UK: The King's Fund; 2015

[18] Lay MM. The Rhetoric of Midwifery: Gender, Knowledge, and Power. New Brunswick, New Jersey and London: Rutgers University Press; 2000

[19] Kantrowitz-Gordon I, Adriane Ellis S, McFarlane A. Men in midwifery: A national survey. Journal of Midwifery & Women's Health. 2014;**59**(5):516-522

[20] Sannomiya M et al. The proportions, regulations, and training plans of male midwives worldwide: A descriptive study of 77 countries. International Journal of Childbirth. 2019;**9**(1):5-18

[21] Muliira RS, Ssendikadiwa VB. Professional quality of life and associated factors among Ugandan midwives working in Mubende and Mityana rural districts. Maternal and Child Health Journal. 2016;**20**:567-576

[22] Allot L, Payne D, Dann L. Midwifery and assisted reproductive technologies. New Zealand College of Midwives Journal. 2013;**47**(47):1, 3, 4

[23] Oelhafen S, Monteverde S, Cignacco E. Exploring moral problems and moral competences in midwifery: A qualitative study. Nursing Ethics. 2019;**26**(5):1373-1386

[24] Rizzo Naudi J. Ethical issues in practice for nurses and midwives: a historical perspective. 2003.

[25] Oelhafen S et al. Increasing midwives' ethical competence: A European educational and practice development project. International Journal of Ethics Education. 2017;**2**:147-160

[26] Sandall J. Midwife-led versus other models of care for childbearing women: Implications of findings from a Cochrane meta-analysis. Evidence-Based Midwifery. 2008;**6**(4):111-112

[27] Homer CS et al. The projected effect of scaling up midwifery. The Lancet. 2014;**384**(9948):1146-1157

[28] Kuipers Y et al. Midwifery-led care: A single mixed-methods synthesis. International Journal of Healthcare Management. 2022;**16**:1-16

[29] Potera C. Evidence supports midwife-led care models. AJN The American Journal of Nursing. 2013;**113**(11):15

[30] Renfrew MJ et al. Midwifery and quality care: Findings from a new evidence-informed framework for maternal and newborn care. The Lancet. 2014;**384**(9948):1129-1145

[31] Shaban I et al. Barriers to developing midwifery as a primary health-care strategy: A Jordanian study. Midwifery. 2012;**28**(1):106-111

[32] Organization WH. Global Strategic Directions for Nursing and Midwifery 2021-2025. 2021.

[33] Jayne Marshall P and A. PGCEA, Approaches to midwifery education. In: Comprehensive Midwifery: The Role of the Midwife in health care practice, education, and Research. 2017.

[34] Chadwick S.C.A.K., Health Needs Assessment-A Practical guide. 2005.

[35] Midwives I.I.C.o., Advocacy. 2023.

[36] Gebresilassie KY et al. Midwifery-led researches for evidence-based practice: Clinical midwives engagement in research in Ethiopia, 2021. PLoS One. 2022;**17**(6):e0268697

[37] Re RN. The role of research in the modern medical Center: The Ochsner clinic foundation perspective. Ochsner Journal. 2006;**6**(1):7-9

Section 3

Mother-Baby Health

Chapter 4

Supporting and Promoting Breastfeeding: The 10 Steps to Successful Breastfeeding

Mary Economou and Nicos Middleton

Abstract

Since the launch of the BFHI (*Baby-Friendly Hospital Initiative*), the "*Ten Steps to Successful Breastfeeding*" have been the cornerstone of national and international strategies that protect and promote breastfeeding. The aim of the BFHI has been the optimization of maternity care services by focusing on the adherence of maternity care facilities to good practices to support and protect breastfeeding. Numerous studies have evaluated the impact of the "10 Steps," employing both observational or intervention study designs, and established higher breastfeeding initiation and longer breastfeeding duration. Nevertheless, suboptimal implementation of the "10 Steps" has been reported in many countries worldwide.

Keywords: breastfeeding, exclusivity, the 10 steps to successful breastfeeding, maternity practices, skin-to-skin, rooming-in

1. Introduction

The joint WHO/UNICEF *Baby-Friendly Hospital Initiative* (BFHI) was launched in 1990 as one of the main components of the Innocenti Declaration on the Protection, Promotion and Support of Breastfeeding. It is an international program which aimed in the improvement of maternity care services, mainly focusing on the adherence of maternity care facilities to "good practices" and specifically the implementation of the "*Ten Steps to Successful Breastfeeding.*" The "10 Steps" are the underpinning of the BFHI and describe the optimal maternity practices for supporting mothers to initiate breastfeeding. The BFHI program was reinvigorated for the first time in 2017 since it was first launched in 1989. The updated implementation guidance targets the policymakers and the institution managers at different levels to fulfill nine responsibilities through a national BFHI program. These are (1) the integration of the 10 Steps into the national policies, (2) establishing or strengthening a national coordination body, (3) ensuring the capacity of all healthcare professionals, (4) the use of external assessment to regularly evaluate the implementation of the 10 Steps, (5) providing technical assistance, (6) monitoring of the implementation, (7) continuous communication and advocacy, (8) identification and allocation of sufficient resources and (9) incentivizing change [1].

IntechOpen

1. Have a written policy that is routinely communicated to all healthcare staff.
2. Train all healthcare staff in the skills necessary to implement this policy.
3. Inform all pregnant women about the benefits and management of breastfeeding.
4. Help mothers initiate breastfeeding within 1 hour of birth.
5. Show mothers how to breastfeed and how to maintain lactation, even if they are separated from their infants.
6. Give infants no food or drink other than breast milk, unless medically indicated.
7. Practice rooming-in—allow mothers and infants to remain together 24 hours a day.
8. Encourage breastfeeding on demand.
9. Give no pacifiers or artificial nipples to breastfeeding infants.
10. Foster the establishment of breastfeeding support groups and refer mothers to them on discharge from the hospital or birth center.
Source: WHO/UNICEF: Baby-Friendly Hospital Initiative: Revised, Updated and Expanded for Integrated Care [2].

Table 1.
The ten steps for successful breastfeeding.

2. BFHI designation and the "ten steps"

A maternity facility is awarded with the designation of Baby-Friendly Hospital when it follows the Global Criteria of the BFHI that were set as the standards for measuring adherence to the 10 Steps for Successful Breastfeeding. The Global Criteria provide guidance on the procedure that maternity care facilities have to undergo in order to be assessed and acquire certification as Baby-Friendly. In 2009, BFHI documents were revised and updated instructions and guidance required for the successful implementation and compliance to the "10 Steps" and the International Code of Marketing of Breast Milk Substitutes were offered [2]. **Table 1** below lists the "10 Steps for Successful Breastfeeding."

A BFHI Self-Appraisal Tool (Section 4) of the ten steps is included in the BFHI package. This tool was developed in order to be used by the maternity care facilities as a means of a preliminary self-assessment of the extent to which they implement the 10 Steps. The self-assessment of maternity care practices which affect successful breastfeeding provides a framework by which a maternity care facility can identify gaps in the implementation to design potential and necessary improvements and modifications. The process follows a triple-A sequence (Assessment, Analysis, and Action). For a maternity facility to acquire the baby-friendly accreditation, it should demonstrate at least 80% compliance to all the maternity practices/Global Criteria as described in the "*Baby-Friendly Hospital Initiative: Revised, Updated and Expanded for Integrated Care*" guide [2]. Accreditation is followed by periodical, predefined re-evaluations to assess to the facility's compliance to the Ten Steps.

3. Current status of the BFHI globally

Since the BFHI was launched, as many as 21,328 maternity care facilities that have been listed as ever been designated as Baby-Friendly in 131 (out of 198; 66%) countries [3]. These represent 27.5% of the all maternity clinics worldwide, ranging from 8.5% in developed countries to 31% in less developed settings [3].

The WHO [4] published an updated report to celebrate the 25th Anniversary since the launch of the initiative. The report provides an analysis of the current status of the BFHI worldwide. Among others, the report describes the global and country program coverage[1], the current designation process as well as reasons of discontinuation of the program in countries that reported its termination. Results of this Report were derived from 2nd Global Nutrition Policy Review (GNPR2), which was distributed to all 194 WHO member states in 2016. The members were requested to ask a series of questions in relation with the implementation of the BFHI. A total of 117 countries completed the questionnaire included in the GNPR2. WHO also obtained information from other sources for countries that did not respond or provided no coverage information to the GNPR2. The additional sources included the 2016 BFHI Network for Industrialized Countries, the 2014 American Health Organization survey on BFHI Implementation in Latin America and the Caribbean, the 2013 UNICEF Nutridash survey. Further, WHO conducted a series of interviews with national leaders in breastfeeding programs and the BFHI in order to receive additional qualitative information of the BFHI [4].

According to the report, 86% of the countries that completed the questionnaire reported that they implemented the BFHI. Overall, 71% reported that they have an operational BFHI program. The BFHI was introduced by almost half (48.8%) of the participating countries in the early 90s, whereas 11 (9.4%) and eight countries (6.8%) have initiated the implementation of BFHI in the period 2000–2009 and 2010–2017 respectively. As many as 16 countries report that they had never implemented the program and for a further 25 countries, the year when the program was actually introduced is not reported [1]. Of the 78 with an active BFHI program that completed the GNPR2 questionnaire, the majority of countries (N = 61; 78%) used the Global Criteria for the assessment of maternity facilities in BFH-designation process. Twenty-one percent (n = 16) used their own national criteria. **Table 2** presents some of the main statistics reported in the Report [4] with regard to the progress and current status of the BFHI countries globally 25 years after the launching of the Initiative.

Table 3 reports the overall percentage of births that occurred in Baby-Friendly-designated hospitals by each WHO region as well as the number of countries per

Year	Number of countries (%)
Never implemented	16 (13.7)
< 1995	34 (29.1)
1995–1999	23 (19.7)
2000–2004	8 (6.8)
2005–2009	3 (2.6)
> 2010	8 (6.8)
Unknown year	25 (21.4)

Source: WHO [1], National Implementation of the Baby-Friendly Hospital Initiative.

Table 2.
Number of countries that reported implementation of the BFHI by year of introduction.

[1] BFHI Coverage is the proportion of births that occur in Baby-Friendly-designated maternity facilities (as defined by the Global Nutrition Monitoring Framework).

Area	% of Births	No of countries on the basis of % BFHI coverage				
		None	< 20%	20–50%	> 50%	Total
Africa	4	15	13	5	2	35
Americas	13	10	16	1	3	30
Easter Mediterranean	17	8	8	4	1	21
Europe	36	16	9	10	12	47
Southeast Asia	3	5	4	0	2	11
Western Pacific	11	9	7	4	4	24
Total	100%	63	57	24	24	168

Source: WHO [1] National Implementation of the Baby-Friendly Hospital Initiative.

Table 3.
Percentage of births that occur in facilities BF-designated maternity facilities by WHO region and number of countries on the basis of the % BFHI coverage.

region on the basis of BFHI coverage (e.g. None through to >50% of births occurring in BFH). Overall, BFHI coverage was estimated at about 10%, ranging from less than 5% in Africa and Southeast Asia to 36% in the European region [4]. However, significant between-country variability is observed, even within the European region. Only 12 (out of 47) countries in the WHO European region report that births in baby-friendly-designated hospitals exceed 50%, whereas as many as 16 countries report of no BF-designated facilities.

Among the participating countries, only 64 have reported that the "10 Steps for Successful Breastfeeding" have been incorporated into national policies or strategies. Only 39 countries (50%) reported having developed a reassessment process. Most of those (N = 21) reassessed the BF maternity facilities less frequently than 5 years and only 14 countries reported that they reassess facilities every 5 years [4].

In 2016, 23 countries reported that they had terminated the implementation of the BFHI. Among those, eight countries ceased its operation before 2005, seven countries stopped the use of the program during the period 2006–2010 and five stopped its implementation within the last 5 years [4]. The most frequently reported reason of BFHI program cessation was the termination of external funding (given by 12 countries), followed by the lack of human resources (given by seven countries), and lack of political interest (given by eight countries). Other reasons mentioned were the termination of governmental funding (given by five countries) and resistance from hospitals or healthcare system (given by five countries). The least common reasons included merging with other programs, lack of advocacy, lack of monitoring and non-adherence of the ICMBS [4].

4. Evidence on the degree of implementation of the "10 steps" and association with breastfeeding

While the original development of the 10 steps was based on clinical experience and good public health practice rather than research evidence in terms of their impact in influencing breastfeeding behavior and outcomes [1], there has been plenty of research evidence since to support the positive association (in observational studies) and/or effectiveness (in intervention studies) of the adherence to BFHI's 10 Steps to Successful Breastfeeding on BF outcomes.

4.1 Degree of implementation of the "10 steps"

Generally, studies conducted to evaluate the impact of Baby-Friendly accredited hospitals demonstrated higher breastfeeding initiation and longer breastfeeding duration [5–7]. However, suboptimal implementation of the "10 Steps" has been reported in many countries worldwide [8–12].

Recording and assessment of the current situation in relation with the implementation of the "10 Steps" in maternity facilities is usually done at a unit level (by the answers provided from the heads/managers of the facilities) and less frequently from the perceived assessment of the facility personnel [13, 14]. The number of studies conducted to investigate the implementation of the Steps through the experiences of mothers seems to be relatively limited [14, 15].

The Maternity Experiences Survey in Canada [12] is one of the largest studies in the literature that assessed the implementation of the 10 steps based on the self-reported experience of a nationally representative sample of over 8000 women, who gave birth during 5–14 months prior to the study. The study reported that the implementation of the 10 steps was fragmented with highest degree of implementation for Step 3 (information about the benefits and management of breastfeeding) and Step 10 where as many as nine out of 10 mothers were given information about where to seek help and support after discharge from the hospital. On the other hand, only one in three mothers experienced skin-to-skin and 44.4% reported that their infant was given a pacifier or a soother within the first week after birth. In a Greek study with the participation of 312 mothers, the majority of the participants (90%) reported that their babies were fed with formula whereas only 3% initiated BF within 1 hour. About 66% of mothers reported rooming-in during their stay in the hospital, of whom all gave birth in a public hospital [9].

4.1.1 Evidence from observational studies

There have been numerous studies from several parts of the world during the last decades that have looked at the association of either the overall implementation (e.g. comparing BF-designated and non-BF-designated hospitals) or partial/select implementation of the 10 steps on BF initiation, duration and exclusivity. Overall, the findings of these studies have consistently demonstrated positive associations of the baby-friendly maternity practices on breastfeeding outcomes.

4.1.2 BF rates in BF-designated and non-BF-designated maternity facilities

This subsection provides evidence of the effect of the BF designation to maternity care facilities (overall effect of the 10 Steps to Successful BF) on BF outcomes. Studies commonly either compared BF and non-BF-designated maternity care facilities [6, 16] or compared changes in select breastfeeding indicators pre- and post-introduction of BF certification [17].

A study [17] that assessed EBF before and after the implementation of the BFHI in a University hospital in Turkey, found that there was a 1.5-fold increase in BF duration with a mean of 21.17 (SD: 0.42) months in the after BFHI group compared to 17.83 (SD: 0.6) months in the pre-BFHI group. Even though the authors found higher EBF rates during the post-BFHI implementation period, the differences were not statistically significant.

In a survey conducted in all Scottish maternity clinics with the inclusion of 464,246 records of infants born during the period of 1995–2002, mothers who gave birth to a Baby-Friendly Hospital were about 28% more likely to initiate breastfeeding within the first week after birth after controlling for the potential effect of confounders [6]. Similar findings have been reported in other studies in terms of initiation [6, 18]. However, unlike breastfeeding initiation, evidence with regard to overall BF duration is conflicting. Whereas several studies have shown a positive effect on BF duration [7, 19], a number of studies did not identify a positive association with longer duration of breastfeeding [16]. For instance, in the Millennium Cohort study in UK with the participation of 17,359 mother-infant dyads from 248 maternity care facilities (of which 14 were BF-designated) higher breastfeeding initiation rates were reported in accredited BFHI hospitals. Nevertheless, this difference was no longer evident by the first month (adj RR: 0.96 95% CI: 0.84, 1.09).

In a different study from the US, with the participation of 29 of a total of 32 BF-designated hospitals, mean breastfeeding initiation rates were significantly higher in comparison to the overall US BF initiation rates (83.8% vs. 69.1%). In addition, mean EBF initiation rates were almost twice higher than the national EBF rates (78.4% vs. 46.3%). Interestingly, the study identified existing inaccuracies in EBF definitions as well as the lack of EBF data recording even in BF-designated hospitals. Only 16 BF hospitals (out of 29 that participated in the study) kept a record of EBF data, and of those only nine reported using the WHO definition for EBF (only breast milk). Six hospitals considered infants to be EBF, even they have also received sugar water for medical reasons and one hospital defined EBF on the basis of maternal perspective on supplementation i.e. infants fed with formula or sugar water for medical reasons were also considered as EBF. According to the hospitals' responses, Steps 3 (*Prenatal Information*), 6 (*only BM*) and 9 (*no use of pacifier or other teats*) were the most difficult to implement. Only a very small number of hospitals, specifically four out of 29, reported no problem on the implementation of the 10 Steps [20].

Implementation of the BFHI also appears to have a positive effect on BF rates in NICUs. Based on extracted data from medical records of infants born and admitted in the NICU of a BF-hospital designated in the USA, in [19]. BF outcomes were compared before the initiation of the procedure for the designation and after the hospital received the certification. The study reported that both BF and EBF initiation as well as duration during the first 6 weeks increased significantly.

4.1.3 Association between the 10 steps and BF outcomes

In a population-based study in the USA, in [21], the five practices that exhibited the strongest association with BF duration within the first 16 weeks independently of maternal socio-economic status, were: (1) initiation of BF within the first hour, (2) only breast milk (exclusive BF), (3) rooming-in, (4) no use of pacifier and (5) BF support after discharge. No association was found between the maternity practices that refer to Hospital staff providing support and information to mothers on breastfeeding (*information given on BF* (step 3); *Help given on how to BF* (Step 5); *BF on Demand* (Step 8); *No gifts or samples of BF substitutes* (ICBS)), suggesting that the type of information and support might not differ. On the contrary, BF duration was higher among mothers that experienced the following steps: *BF within the first hour after birth* (Step 4); *only BM while in the maternity clinic* (Step 6); *Rooming-in* (Step 7);

No use of a pacifier (Step 9) compared to those that they did not. When the effect of the implementation of the five maternity practices was investigated on the basis of their socio-economic status (defined as mothers whose incomes <= 185% of the poverty level and those whose incomes were > 185 the poverty level), low-income mothers reported higher BF rates between 1 and 14 weeks among those that experienced all five maternity clinics compared to those that did not (65% vs. 46%). For mothers above >185 the poverty level, BF rates among those that experience all maternity practices were significantly higher than those that did not between 9 and 12 weeks (at 12 weeks: 82% vs. 70%).

In a longitudinal study (Infant Feeding Practices Survey) conducted in the USA [22], five indicators were measured, thought to negatively affect breastfeeding outcomes to reflect the lack of implementation of good maternity care practices as described in the 10 steps, namely late BF initiation, introduction of supplementation, not rooming-in, not breastfeeding on demand, use of pacifiers. These were directly assessed by mothers who initiated breastfeeding during their stay in the maternity clinic and expressed the intention to BF for at least 2 months during pregnancy. The findings suggested a clear dose-response relationship between maternity practices and the risk of BF discontinuation before the first 6 weeks of birth. In fact, the fewer the number of "good practices" the mothers experienced during their stay, the higher the risk of BF discontinuation. Specifically, mothers who reported that they did no experience any of the maternity practices were nearly eight times more likely to discontinue BD prematurely by comparison to those who reported experienced all of the above five practices/steps (adjOR: 7.7; 95% CI: 2.3–25.8). When each "bad practice" was assessed separately, three of the five steps appeared to be more strongly associated with shorter BF duration; late BF initiation, supplementation and no BF on demand. After adjustment for other variables, late BF initiation and supplementation were identified as the stronger risk factors of early BF discontinuation. Mothers who experienced none of the maternity practices were about seven times more likely to discontinue BF within the first 6 weeks in comparison to those experienced all five practices. Among the factors that were found to be independently associated with discontinuation of BF before the sixth week were Initiation of breastfeeding (adj OR: 1.6; 95% CI: 1.1–2.3); formula supplementation (adj OR: 2.3; 95% CI: 1.5–3.3) and not BF on demand (adj OR: 1.2; 95% CI: 0.8–1.7). On the other hand, pacifier use (adj OR: 1.0; 95% CI: 0.7–1.4) and rooming-in (adj OR: 1.1; 95% CI: 0.8–1.7) were found not to be associated with BF discontinuation.

While there is clear evidence to suggest that the use of supplementation is one of the strongest independent risk factors of exclusivity as well as shorter BF duration in general, it has been suggested that even baby-friendly-designated hospitals fail to achieve its implementation. The Baby-Friendly requirement that the maternity clinics have to pay for the infant formulas, especially in countries that hospitals receive formulas from the companies for free, increases significantly the maternity clinics' expenses and becomes a barrier to the adherence of Step 6 (*Only BM*) [5].

A Swiss study [23] also confirmed the positive association between the implementation of BFHI and exclusivity as well as longer breastfeeding duration. While an improvement in BF and EBF rates was observed after accreditation of hospitals with the baby-friendly designation during 1994–2004, the authors observed significant variability in EBF rates as well as the degree of meeting the BFHI criteria, even among hospitals that acquired the designation. In the study, the authors reported that the strongest associations with shorter BF duration were observed in terms of formula supplementation in the maternity facility. Moreover, the introduction of other liquids (not formula supplementation) was also associated with early cessation of BF. BF within the first hour after birth, full rooming-in, breastfeeding on demand and no use of pacifiers was shown to be associated with longer BF and EBF duration.

A survey in Brazil [24], as part of an immunization campaign, included 65,936 infants younger than 1 year of age and examined the association of the implementation of Baby-Friendly practices on breastfeeding outcomes. A higher proportion of mothers who delivered in a Baby-Friendly Hospital were more likely to experience the 10 steps. The experience of the 10 steps was shown to have a positive association with the duration of EBF up to the sixth month. Similar findings are confirmed by a series of studies from other countries [25, 26]. It has been suggested, however, that mothers who intend to BF longer or exclusively are more likely to choose to give birth in a Baby-Friendly hospital and are more willing to comply with the 10 Steps; hence, to some extent to which the observed differences represent a selection bias is not clear [26].

In any case, there is evidence to suggest that any effect is likely to be cumulative as the more "good practices" mothers experience the more likely they are to achieve EBF intentions [27]. Findings from the Infant Feeding study II in the USA suggest that experiencing all six practices investigated [*Initiate BF within 1 hour after birth* (Step 4); *only breast milk* (Step 6); *Rooming-In* (Step 7); *BF on Demand* (Step 8); *Use no Pacifier/Teats* (Step 9); *Provide information on how to seek support after discharge* (Step 10)] increases the odds of achieving the mother's intended duration of EBF by nearly three times in comparison to experiencing none or only one [27]. Furthermore, compared to mothers who experienced all six baby-friendly practices, mother that had not experienced any of the practices were at 13 times greater risk to discontinue any BF [8]. As additional baby-friendly practices were implemented, a stepwise decrease of the risk was observed, suggesting a dose–response relationship between the number of the Steps and breastfeeding. Using logistic regression analysis in order to implement mutual adjustment between the maternity practices [(*BF initiation within 1 hour* (Step 4); *only BM given* (Step 6), *Rooming-in* (Step 7), *BF on Demand* (Step 8); *No pacifiers given* (Step 9); *Provide information on BF* (Step 10) as well as to adjust for several socio-demographic factors (e.g. child gender, household income, marital status, parity, maternal education) and behavioral and attitudinal factors [e.g. number of friends and relatives who breastfed, maternal prenatal intentions to work after birth, prenatal attitudes toward BF (i.e. formula as good as BM)], the authors identified the three practices with the strongest positive association with BF outcomes in the first 6 weeks period after birth. These are: BF initiation within 1 hour, only breast milk given and no pacifiers or other soothers.

Another study [28] conducted in four Public hospitals in Hong Kong with a sample of 1242 mother-infant pairs investigated the effect of six maternity practices on breastfeeding duration up to the first month after birth. The maternity practices not investigated were: *Have a written BF policy* (Step 1), *Train health workers to implement the policy* (Step 2), *Inform all pregnant women about the benefits and management of BF* (Step 3) and *Support mothers on how to BF* (Step 5). Mothers who did not experience any of the good maternity care practices were about three times more likely to initiate weaning within the first 8 weeks (AdjOR: 3.13; 95% CI: 1.41–6.95). In order to identify the practices that are more strongly associated with successful breastfeeding outcomes, the authors performed a multivariable analysis. Only four of the six maternity practices investigated were associated with BF discontinuation at 8 weeks after adjustment for socio-demographic factors, mode of birth, return to work and other breastfeeding support factors. These are early BF initiation within 1 hour after birth (AdjOR: 0.65; 95% CI: 0.51–0.83), only breast milk (AdjOR: 0.47; 95% CI: 0.35–0.63), no use of a pacifier (AdjOR: 0.66; 95% CI: 0.53–0.83), breastfeeding information and support (AdjOR: 0.67; 95% CI: 0.52–0.88). The study did not find any association between rooming-in (AdjOR: 1.13; 95% CI: 0.89–1.43) and breastfeeding on demand (AdjOR: 1.01; 95% CI: 0.78–1.31) and BF duration. When in the multivariate model, breastfeeding support variables (whether the mother BF as an infant, previous BF experience and paternal preference to BF) were also included, only EBF while in hospital stay (Step 6) was associated with BF duration.

It has to be noted that the majority of studies operationalize the extent to which the "10 steps" have been implemented based on self-report of the mothers. Furthermore, even though the set of good practices refers to 10 items, the first two items (i.e. written policy and education of maternity clinic staff) are almost always never included in the investigation since these are clinic-level rather than individual-level variables and, unlike other steps (for example, breastfeeding within 1 hour of birth, rooming-in, breastfeeding on demand and so on) cannot be reported by the participating mothers in the form of self-reported experience.

A prospective study by Pincombe et al. [11] with a sample of 317 primiparous mothers in Australia followed for the first 6 months after birth found that the use of formula supplementation, the use of pacifier/dummy or nipple shield and, interestingly, breastfeeding on demand while in the hospital were associated with shorter duration of breastfeeding. After adjusting for different socio-demographic factors, "breastfeeding on demand" remained positively associated with early initiation of weaning (adjHR: 1.71; 95% CI: 1.03–2.86). The authors concluded that the surprising association between breastfeeding on demand and shorter duration of breastfeeding was confounded by other factors such as higher self-efficacy, smoking less, education level, type of birth delivery [11].

Even though studies have varied in terms of their study design (set of steps included in the investigation, breastfeeding outcomes, length of follow-up and so on), it appears that the most consistent, and perhaps non-surprising, association with early discontinuation of exclusive breastfeeding is the provision of other non-breast milk liquids while at the clinic [11, 27], especially formula supplementation [29–31].

A US national study [32] examined the effect of the implementation of the 10 Steps for mothers to achieve their intention for EBF duration in primiparas and multiparas separately. For primiparas, four maternity practices were associated with BF intention: only breast milk (not other supplement) (adjOR: 4.4; 95% CI: 2.1–9.3), providing information on community BF support resources (adjOR: 2.3; 95% CI: 1.1–4.9); health support for BF initiation (adjOR: 6.3; 95% CI: 1.8–21.6); no use of pacifier (adjOR: 2.3; 95% CI: 1.1–4.4). For multiparas, only breast milk (adjOR: 8.8; 95% CI: 4.4–17.6) and support of BF on demand (adjOR: 3.4; 95% CI: 1.7–6.8) were the only maternity services that were statistically significant with the fulfillment of the maternal intention of EBF duration.

4.2 Evidence from intervention studies

The majority of studies assessing the association between the implementation of the "10 steps" and breastfeeding outcomes in the published literature are observational. This was also the conclusion of a systematic review on the subject [33]. Of 58 reports identified in their review, nine were based on three randomized controlled trials. The rest of the studies were quasi-experimental designs (N = 19), prospective studies (N = 11) and cross-sectional or retrospective (N = 19). Even so, the authors concluded that adherence to the Ten Steps has a positive impact on short-term, medium-term and long-term breastfeeding outcomes with a dose-response relationship between the number of steps and the likelihood of improved BF outcomes. Interestingly, they also concluded that community support (step 10) appears to be essential for sustaining any impacts of the BFHI in the long term. The lack of intervention studies is not surprising due to the nature of the intervention and the pragmatic difficulty in randomizing units to BFHI. It is more likely that studies apply observational designs either in the form of descriptive comparative designs i.e. comparing maternity units that have implemented the BFHI to control facilities [34] or pre-post quasi-experimental designs [35, 36]. These studies have been discussed in the section above alongside the observational studies with a survey study design.

The first intervention study was the seminal and most well-cited to date PROBIT study in the Republic of Belarus [34]. This was a cluster randomized trial. The study investigated the effectiveness of BFHI by randomly assigning 31 hospitals to either the BFHI intervention or control arm. During the study period, as many as 17.046 mother-infant dyads were included in the data analysis. The prevalence of Breastfeeding and Exclusive Breastfeeding was measured at 3, 6, 9 and 12 months. The study found a higher prevalence of BF in the maternity clinics in the intervention arm compared to the control arm at the third (72.7% vs. 60%; adjOR: 0.52, 95% CI: 0.40, 0.69) and sixth month of follow-up (49.8% vs. 36.1%; adjOR: 0.52, 95% CI: 0.39, 0.71). Furthermore, the study showed differences between intervention-control arm at longer follow-up periods. The breastfeeding prevalence at 9 months among the group of women who delivered in a BFHI hospital (intervention arm) was 36.1% in comparison to 24.2% among mothers who gave birth in the control hospitals (adjOR: 0.51, 95% CI: 0.36, 0.73). At 12 months, the prevalence of BF was 19.7% in the intervention group compared to 11.4% in the control group (adjOR: 0.47, 95% CI: 0.32, 0.69).

The study demonstrated that the effectiveness of the implementation of the BFHI on improving breastfeeding was not short-lived since differences between intervention and control arms were observed both in the short term as well as the long term, and up to a period of 12 months after birth. Furthermore, the study found that the effect was not just restricted to a higher likelihood and longer duration of any breastfeeding, but also showed a significant effect of the intervention on exclusive breastfeeding. The proportion of mothers exclusively breastfeeding at 3 months was seven times higher in the experimental group than the control group (43.3% vs. 6.4%; p-value<0.001) and more than 12 times higher at 6 months after birth (7.9% vs. 0.6%; p-value = 0.01). Of course, it should be noted that even though there was a statistically significant effect of the intervention on the likelihood of breastfeeding at 6 months after birth (49.8% vs. 36.1% in the control group), as well as the likelihood that this is exclusive by comparison to the control group, the prevalence of mothers who exclusively breastfed at 6 months was quite low even in the intervention arm (7.9% vs. 0.6%). This finding is not surprising since recommendations for EBF are for 6 months.

The other two intervention studies identified by a review [33] were conducted in Brazil. However, the aim was not to assess the BFHI 10 steps as a pack, but certain aspects of it. In a study [37], following training of the maternity care staff in the 10 steps, mothers were randomized to receive 10 postnatal home visits (step 10). The authors found that strengthening step 10 had a significant positive impact of the intervention on the prevalence of exclusive and any breastfeeding. Taddei et al. [35] randomly assigned eight hospitals in Brazil to Ten Steps training or to continue the standard of care but did not find an impact of the training of the staff on breastfeeding duration.

A quasi-experimental study [36] was conducted in the USA with the participation of 13 hospitals that received BF accreditation before 1999 or became accredited during the period 1999–2009 (participants = 11,723) and 19 non-BF-designated matched hospitals (participants = 136,040). Matching was achieved by identifying the Baby-Friendly maternity facility's "nearest neighbors," determined by calculating the Euclidian distance between standardized values of pairs of observations. These were the number of births as a proxy for the size of birth facility, the proportion of white mothers and the proportion of mothers with high education. Even though the study did not find an overall difference between the BF and non-BF-designated hospitals, the study reported a differential effect of the intervention in terms of educational attainment. In fact, the study recorded an increase of 3.8% in Breastfeeding initiation rates in designated Baby-friendly hospitals (adj coef = 0.038; 95% CI: 0.00, 0.08) and of 4.5% in EBF for 4 months or more (adj coeff = 0.045; 95% CI: 0.01, 0.08) for only among mothers of lower educational attainment. This is due to the fact that mothers with higher maternal education are more likely to be aware of the BF accreditation and thereafter choose to give birth in Baby-friendly hospitals. On the contrary, BF accreditation might help to reduce the effect of socio-economic disparities and therefore reduce the gap of health inequalities. Similar were the findings by Sherburne-Hawkins et al. [38] with the participation of a smaller number of BFHI (n = 4, participants = 915) and non-BFHI hospitals (n = 6, participants = 1099) with an increase of 8.6% in Breastfeeding initiation rates in designated Baby-friendly hospitals (adj coeff: 0.086; 95% CI: 0.01–0.16) only among mothers of lower educational attainment. Also, for each additional BF maternity practice, there was an increase in BF initiation (adj coeff, 0.146 [95% CI, 0.13–0.16).

5. Summary

For over two decades, the "10 Steps" have been the cornerstone of national and international policies and strategies for the promotion, protection and support of BF. However, adherence to the "10 Steps" is suboptimal [10, 12, 22]. In fact, it seems that the maternity care practices which are more consistently associated with a positive impact on BF [22] appear to be the least implemented, such as the practice of early initiation of breastfeeding in skin-to-skin position and no use of a pacifier [12].

The literature that supports the beneficial effects of the adherence to the BFHI on BF outcomes, and specifically "good maternity care practices" in the model of the "10 Steps," is extensive. Observational and intervention studies have assessed the impact of implementation of the "10 Steps" on BF outcomes and have consistently shown positive effects on BF initiation, duration and exclusivity. The effect of the "10 Steps" is also apparent in the reduction of social inequalities in BF.

However, evidence of the individual effect of the "10 Steps" on BF outcomes is conflicting. While the implementation of specific maternity care practices has been consistently associated with BF outcomes, evidence is not as consistent or clear-cut for others. For example, immediate and longer skin-to-skin has been associated with higher BF initiation rates [39] as well as longer EBF and BF duration [40, 41]. Similarly, implementation of Step 9 (no pacifiers) has been acknowledged to be associated with longer BF [42–44] and EBF duration [45]. However, pacifier use might represent an outcome of a rather complex maternal behavior which is difficult to pinpoint. For instance, mothers who do not intent to breastfeed, encounter lactation problems or decide to discontinue BF are more likely to introduce a pacifier as a result.

Thus, the direction of the association between pacifier use and breastfeeding is not clear. In relation to Step 3 (education in the prenatal period), evidence on the effect of breastfeeding initiation and duration is also not clear. While a number of studies suggest a beneficial effect of prenatal information on BF outcomes, others do not [21]. The type and nature of the interventions seem to influence the effectiveness of Step 3 on BF outcomes.

Author details

Mary Economou and Nicos Middleton*
Cyprus University of Technology, Limassol, Cyprus

*Address all correspondence to: nicos.middleton@cut.ac.cy

References

[1] WHO. National Hospital Initiative of the Baby-Friendly Implementation 2017. 2017. Available from: http://apps.who.int/iris/bitstream/10665/255197/1/9789241512381-eng.pdf?ua=1 [Accessed: March, 2023]

[2] WHO. Section 4: Hospital Self-Appraisal and Monitoring. Baby-Friendly Hospital Initiative: Revised, Updated and Expanded for Integrated Care. Geneva, Switzerland: World Health Organization; 2009. Available from: https://www.unicef.org/nutrition/files/BFHI_2009_s4.pdf [Accessed: May, 2023]

[3] Labbok MH. Global baby-friendly hospital initiative monitoring data: Update and discussion. Breastfeeding Medicine. 2012;7(4):210-222

[4] WHO. National Implementation of the Baby-Friendly Hospital Initiative. 2017. Available from: http://apps.who.int/iris/bitstream/handle/10665/255197/9789241512381-eng.pdf?sequence=1 [Accessed: March, 2023]

[5] Philipp BL, Merewood A, Miller LW, Chawla N, Murphy-Smith MM, Gomes JS, et al. Baby-friendly hospital initiative improves breastfeeding initiation rates in a US hospital setting. Pediatrics. 2001;**108**(3):677-681

[6] Broadfoot M, Britten J, Tappin DM, MacKenzie JM. The baby friendly hospital initiative and breast feeding rates in Scotland. Archives of Disease in Childhood-Fetal and Neonatal Edition. 2005;**90**(2):F114-F116

[7] Brodribb W, Kruske S, Miller YD. Baby-friendly hospital accreditation, in-hospital care practices, and breastfeeding. Pediatrics. 2013;**131**(4):685-692

[8] DiGirolamo AM, Grummer-Strawn LM, Fein SB. Effect of maternity-care practices on breastfeeding. Pediatrics. 2008;**122**(Supplement 2):S43-S49

[9] Theofilogiannakou M, Skouroliakou M, Gounaris A, Panagiotakos D, Markantonis SL. Breast-feeding in Athens, Greece: Factors associated with its initiation and duration. Journal of Pediatric Gastroenterology and Nutrition. 2006;**43**(3):379-384

[10] Chien LY, Tai CJ, Chu KH, Ko YL, Chiu YC. The number of baby friendly hospital practices experienced by mothers is positively associated with breastfeeding: A questionnaire survey. International Journal of Nursing Studies. 2007;**44**(7):1138-1146

[11] Pincombe J, Baghurst P, Antoniou G, Peat B, Henderson A, Reddin E. Baby friendly hospital initiative practices and breast feeding duration in a cohort of first-time mothers in Adelaide, Australia. Midwifery. 2008;**24**(1):55-61

[12] Chalmers B, Levitt C, Heaman M, O'brien B, Sauve R, Kaczorowski J; Maternity Experiences Study Group of the Canadian Perinatal Surveillance System, Public Health Agency of Canada.Breastfeeding rates and hospital breastfeeding practices in Canada: A national survey of women. Birth. 2009;**36**(2):122-132

[13] Grizzard TA, Bartick M, Nikolov M, Griffin BA, Lee KG. Policies and practices related to breastfeeding in Massachusetts: Hospital implementation of the ten steps to successful breastfeeding. Maternal and Child Health Journal. 2006;**10**(3):247-263

[14] Haiek LN. Compliance with baby-friendly policies and practices in hospitals and community health centers in Quebec. Journal of Human Lactation. 2012;**28**(3):343-358

[15] Abul-Fadl AM, Shawky M, El-Taweel A, Cadwell K, Turner-Maffei C. Evaluation of mothers' knowledge, attitudes, and practice towards the ten steps to successful breastfeeding in Egypt. Breastfeeding Medicine. 2012;**7**(3):173-178

[16] Bartington S, Griffiths LJ, Tate AR, Dezateux C. Are breastfeeding rates higher among mothers delivering in baby friendly accredited maternity units in the UK? International Journal of Epidemiology. 2006;**35**(5):1178-1186

[17] Duyan Camurdan A, Özkan S, Yüksel D, Pasli F, Şahin F, Beyazova U. The effect of the baby-friendly hospital initiative on long-term breast feeding. International Journal of Clinical Practice. 2007;**61**(8):1251-1255

[18] Mydlilova A, Sipek A, Vignerova J. Breastfeeding rates in baby-friendly and non-baby-friendly hospitals in the Czech Republic from 2000 to 2006. Journal of Human Lactation. 2009;**25**(1):73-78

[19] Merewood A, Philipp BL, Chawla N, Cimo S. The baby-friendly hospital initiative increases breastfeeding rates in a US neonatal intensive care unit. Journal of Human Lactation. 2003;**19**(2):166-171

[20] Merewood A, Mehta SD, Chamberlain LB, Philipp BL, Bauchner H. Breastfeeding rates in US baby-friendly hospitals: Results of a national survey. Pediatrics. 2005;**116**(3):628-634

[21] Murray EK, Ricketts S, Dellaport J. Hospital practices that increase breastfeeding duration: Results from a population-based study. Birth. 2007;**34**(3):202-211

[22] DiGirolamo AM, Grummer-Strawn LM, Fein S. Maternity care practices: Implications for breastfeeding. Birth. 2001;**28**(2):94-100

[23] Merten S, Ackermann-Liebrich U. Exclusive breastfeeding rates and associated factors in Swiss baby-friendly hospitals. Journal of Human Lactation. 2004;**20**(1):9-17

[24] Venancio SI, Saldiva SRDM, Escuder MML, Giugliani ERJ. The baby-friendly hospital initiative shows positive effects on breastfeeding indicators in Brazil. Journal of Epidemiology and Community Health. 2011;(10):jech-2011

[25] Braun MLG, Giugliani ER, Soares MEM, Giugliani C, de Oliveira AP, Danelon CMM. Evaluation of the impact of the baby-friendly hospital initiative on rates of breastfeeding. American Journal of Public Health. 2003;**93**(8):1277-1279

[26] Merten S, Dratva J, Ackermann-Liebrich U. Do baby-friendly hospitals influence breastfeeding duration on a national level? Pediatrics. 2005;**116**(5):e702-e708

[27] Perrine CG, Scanlon KS, Li R, Odom E, Grummer-Strawn LM. Baby-friendly hospital practices and meeting exclusive breastfeeding intention. Pediatrics. 2012;**130**(1):54-60

[28] Tarrant M, Wu KM, Fong DY, Lee IL, Wong EM, Sham A, et al. Impact of baby-friendly hospital practices on breastfeeding in Hong Kong. Birth. 2011;**38**(3):238-245

[29] Parry JE, Ip DK, Chau PY, Wu KM, Tarrant M. Predictors and consequences of in-hospital formula supplementation for healthy breastfeeding newborns. Journal of Human Lactation. 2013;**29**(4):527-536

[30] Semenic S, Loiselle C, Gottlieb L. Predictors of the duration of exclusive breastfeeding among first-time mothers. Research in Nursing and Health. 2008;**31**(5):428-441

[31] Chantry CJ, Dewey KG, Peerson JM, Wagner EA, Nommsen-Rivers LA. In-hospital formula use increases early breastfeeding cessation among first-time mothers intending to exclusively breastfeed. The Journal of Pediatrics. 2014;**164**(6):1339-1345

[32] Declercq E, Labbok MH, Sakala C, O'hara M. Hospital practices and women's likelihood of fulfilling their intention to exclusively breastfeed. American Journal of Public Health. 2009;**99**(5):929-935

[33] Pérez-Escamilla R, Martinez JL, Segura-Pérez S. Impact of the baby-friendly hospital initiative on breastfeeding and child health outcomes: A systematic review. Maternal & Child Nutrition. 2016;**12**(3):402-417

[34] Kramer MS, Chalmers B, Hodnett ED, Sevkovskaya Z, Dzikovich I, Shapiro S, et al. Promotion of breastfeeding intervention trial (PROBIT): A randomized trial in the Republic of Belarus. JAMA. 2001;**285**(4):413-420

[35] Taddei JADAC, Westphal MF, Venancio S, Bogus C, Souza S. Breastfeeding training for health professionals and resultant changes in breastfeeding duration. Sao Paulo Medical Journal. 2000;**118**(6):185-191

[36] Hawkins SS, Stern AD, Baum CF, Gillman MW. Evaluating the impact of the baby-friendly hospital initiative on breast-feeding rates: A multi-state analysis. Public Health Nutrition. 2015;**18**(2):189-197

[37] Coutinho SB, de Lira PIC, de Carvalho Lima M, Ashworth A. Comparison of the effect of two systems for the promotion of exclusive breastfeeding. The Lancet. 2005;**366**(9491):1094-1100

[38] Hawkins SS, Stern AD, Baum CF, Gillman MW. Compliance with the Baby-Friendly Hospital initiative and impact on breastfeeding rates. Archives of Disease in Childhood-Fetal and Neonatal Edition. 2014;**99**(2):F138-F143

[39] Asole S, Spinelli A, Antinucci LE, Di Lallo D. Effect of hospital practices on breastfeeding: A survey in the Italian Region of Lazio. Journal of Human Lactation. 2009;**25**(3):333-340

[40] Mikiel-Kostyra K, Mazur J, Boltruszko I. Effect of early skin-to-skin contact after delivery on duration of breastfeeding: A prospective cohort study. Acta Paediatrica. 2002;**91**(12):1301-1306

[41] Bramson L, Lee JW, Moore E, Montgomery S, Neish C, Bahjri K, et al. Effect of early skin-to-skin mother—infant contact during the first 3 hours following birth on exclusive breastfeeding during the maternity hospital stay. Journal of Human Lactation. 2010;**26**(2):130-137

[42] Howard CR, Howard FM, Lanphear B, Eberly S, Lawrence RA. The effects of early pacifier use on breastfeeding duration. Pediatrics. 1999;**103**(3):e33-e33

[43] O'Connor NR, Tanabe KO, Siadaty MS, Hauck FR. Pacifiers and breastfeeding: A systematic review. Archives of Pediatrics & Adolescent Medicine. 2009;**163**(4):378-382

[44] Aarts C, Hörnell A, Kylberg E, Hofvander Y, Gebre-Medhin M. Breastfeeding patterns in relation to thumb sucking and pacifier use. Pediatrics. 1999;**104**(4):e50-e50

[45] de Nascimento MBR, Reis MAM, Franco SC, Issler H, Ferraro AA, Grisi SJF. Exclusive breastfeeding in southern Brazil: Prevalence and associated factors. Breastfeeding Medicine. 2010;**5**(2):79-85

Chapter 5

Description of a Relationship Focused Mother-Infant Group Program: Mother-Baby Nurture

Sharon Cooke, Dawson Cooke and Sue Coleson

Abstract

Mother-Baby Nurture is an innovative group program that focusses on strengthening the mother-infant relationship through enhancing reflective capacity within mothers and their infants. We describe the unique combination of the features that are central to this program and present comparisons with other early parenting interventions. Infancy is a unique period of acute developmental vulnerability and dependence on a caregiver. As the caregiver is the critical regulator between infant and their environment, disturbances in the caregiver-infant relationship have heightened potential to interfere in the infant's developmental trajectory and lifelong wellbeing. Mother-Baby Nurture is a 10-week targeted group program that is currently being implemented in Western Australia, for infants and their mothers experiencing relational or emotional distress. This program provides an emotionally containing space for a mother and her infant to explore mental states. We foster curiosity in the thoughts, feelings, and behaviour (of the baby, the mother, and others), as well as reflection on attachment relationships (past and present). This therapeutic approach shares common ground with parent-infant psychotherapy and mentalization-based treatment, and is informed by attachment theory and the neurobiological science of infant development.

Keywords: Mother-Baby Nurture, group, infant, mother, relationship, parenting, mentalization-based treatment

1. Introduction

Early infancy, more than any other time in the human lifecycle, is a time of unprecedented developmental capacity and vulnerability. During this time, experiences powerfully influence brain architecture and subsequently provide the foundation for all future learning [1, 2]. Adverse early experiences during the formative months of infancy, if not addressed, can have lifelong consequences for the developing person [3] and can be transmitted the next generation [4]. A critical experience during infancy is the relationship with caregivers, and for most infants the relationship with their mother is particularly influential.

In 1940, Winnicott declared "there is no such thing as an infant [on his or her own]", the infant exists "as a unit" in relationship with a caregiver [5]. Bowlby [6] described how ideally, the caregiver-infant relationship provides the infant with a secure base from which they can explore the world and return to have their needs met. A central means by which a parent influences the security of their relationship with their child is the capacity of mentalizing [7]; also referred to as reflective functioning [8]. Parental mentalizing helps the infant to make sense of their 'self' and their external world, as the caregiver provides a conduit for sharing, understanding, and regulating internal mental states including thoughts, feelings, longings, and desires. The capacity to mentalize and provide this secure base for the infant may be distorted or enabled by the caregiver's organisation of their own past childhood experiences of their caregivers, that informs their internal working model [9]. The transmission of secure infant-caregiver attachment across the generations provides the context for optimal psychological, social and emotional development of the infant, and is predictive of future social-emotional and cognitive functioning throughout the early years and into adulthood [10, 11]. This premise, that social, emotional and cognitive development during infancy occurs within the context of the infant-caregiver relationship, is an anchor point for the field of infant mental health [12], psychodynamic early intervention [13], and the central rationale behind Mother-Baby Nurture (MBN).

We provide a description of the MBN program and the nuanced role of the group facilitators. Following this is a discussion of the key distinguishing concepts at the heart of MBN: the importance of early relational experiences, infant as participant, the group as a containing space, and enhancing mentalizing [14]. The outcomes anticipated for the mother and for the infant are reflected upon. In this discussion paper, caregivers are described as 'she', and for ease of reading, infants will be described as 'he'.

2. Description of Mother-Baby Nurture program

Mother-Baby Nurture is a brief reflective group program for mothers and their infants (0–6 months of age) facilitated by two infant mental health clinicians over a 10-week duration in a community setting. Weekly 2-hour sessions take place with the facilitators and six mothers forming the outer circle, with babies held in mother's arms or within reach on baby rugs in the circle centre. It is an experiential group, where the pace is slow and spacious, and responsive to the felt needs of the babies and their mothers. Together, we agree on group guidelines to help create a safe space, where mothers and babies are invited to take time getting to know one another. There are predictable weekly rituals that invite curiosity, observation, and reflection. These include the mother-baby check-in, watch-with-wonder, infant observation time, nursery rhymes, and the use of imagery, metaphors, poetry, and music. The rituals are offered as gentle entry points for reflective discussion. Dedicated attachment-relationship themes are introduced and explored in an effort to bring to mind past and present patterns of relating. Reflecting on mother-infant interaction helps to illuminate patterns of relating that may not have been previously noticed or thought about. Throughout the group, the infants' communications are welcomed, held in mind, and responded to, which significantly shapes the content and pace of the group process.

The primary intervention aim of MBN is to strengthen the mother-infant relationship. A central strategy to improve the relationship and infant outcomes is to foster and strengthen the mother's mentalizing capacity. A secondary strategy of the program is the reduction of symptoms of maternal postnatal depression and anxiety as well improving the mothers' parenting confidence and feelings of attachment with their infant [15].

We acknowledge that every family exists within the context of broader caregiving systems, with unique family, community and cultural expectations and structures [16]. Issues highlighted in the mother-infant relationship may also be relevant to father-infant relationships or other caregivers and family system level relationships [17, 18], although these dynamics are beyond the scope of this paper. In response to community demand, this program has been adapted for the unique needs of Aboriginal, culturally and linguistically diverse as well as adolescent mothers and their families. Presently, MBN is provided at ten locations across Western Australia, delivering 40 10-week groups per year, servicing approximately 240 vulnerable families every year.

2.1 Role of the MBN facilitators

Facilitators are recruited from different disciplines including psychology, social work, counselling, midwifery, and other relevant fields of allied health. Each facilitator has undertaken a three-day manualised MBN training process [14] and participates in ongoing monthly reflective supervision. Each group has a lead and co-facilitator, and over time through the process of mentoring, the co-facilitator may become the lead facilitator when the opportunity arises. Reflective supervision is a vital ingredient when working with young children and their caregivers in the shared exploration of the emotional content [19, 20]. Reflective supervision offers an emotionally containing relationship that mirrors the role of the facilitator with the mothers; this is vital to keep the thinking and feeling alive on behalf of the group. The main focus of this supervision is "the shared exploration of the emotional content of infant and family work as expressed in relationships between parents and infants, parents and practitioners, and supervisors and practitioners" [21, p. 63].

The role of the MBN facilitators is to create an emotionally containing environment for the mothers and infants while making mentalizing explicit through maintaining a stance of curiosity and reflection. The facilitator holds the baby in mind as a separate being whose experience and behaviours are meaningful while holding the mother's experience, even though these may seem intolerable or distorted at times [22]. To sufficiently hold the powerful projections and primitive processes in the mother-baby group, two facilitators are recommended [23].

The facilitators narrate their observations aloud in the group, at times making sense of differences of perspective, modelling not knowing the other's mind as well as sharing co-joint intent to work together to support group members [24, 25]. There may be minor misunderstandings and differences in the facilitator's perspectives, and these distinctions are talked about to model "good enough" parent relationship to the mothers. Facilitators may stop and rewind, slow the pace or seek clarification in an effort to reflect upon a shared moment when a member responds in a particular way. Emotional reactions are noted; sometimes explicitly identified and explored, perhaps acknowledged and explored at a later time, or simply noted for facilitators' shared reflection after the group. We acknowledge and celebrate moments of attunement and delight as well as offering a kind and curious presence in moments of distress and mis-attunement. As the facilitators work together in an unhurried pace, thinking aloud about the affects and processes encountered in the group, whilst holding each member in mind, they attempt to embody the qualities found in a collaborative parenting model for the members to experience [23]. Facilitators work together to support one another to develop a reflective stance and to help provide a clearer lens to observe group processes and model mentalizing as a way of being together. In addition, co-facilitation can represent alternate perspectives, such as a father's experience or other siblings [23].

On becoming a mother, a woman's relationship with her own mother may be thrown into sharp relief, with mixed and often ambivalent feelings surfacing unexpectedly. In the MBN group setting, the facilitators may find the mothers relating to them in ways that echo these ambivalences. By maintaining consistent, thoughtful, compassionate, and accepting stance, facilitators offer a potentially new experience for mothers where these qualities may have been longed-for but not experienced in their relationship with their own caregivers. Once experienced, these mothers may become able to draw on an internal representations of a 'good grandmother' [26] facilitator to help contain and make sense of thoughts and feelings in a new and enriched way.

3. Key distinguishing concepts of MBN

There are four key concepts that we have identified as underpinning the Mother-Baby Nurture model: early relational experiences matter, infant as participant, the group as a containing space, and enhancing mentalizing.

3.1 Early relational experiences matter

The first six months post birth is a time of profound transition for both infant and mother. It is a highly sensitive period in the newborn infant's neurobiological development whereby exposure to early stressful experiences (such as an emotionally dysregulated mother) may alter the developing hypothalamic pituitary adrenal (HPA - stress response) system, sensitising the individual to future stressful life events and psychopathology [27]. It is also a vulnerable period of neuropsychological development where repeated relational experiences between mother and infant, over time accumulate to inform the infant's internal working model, shaping the patterns of attachment behaviour in response to the mother [2, 28]. The quality of these early attachments is understood to contribute significantly to a child's long term socio-emotional development [29].

Described by Stern [26] as the "motherhood constellation", the presence of the infant typically activates the mother's attachment system, preoccupying the mother's mind and body with the survival and nurture of her baby. It can be an intense period of psychological reorganisation that may involve reshaping of the mother's perceived role, identity, internal working model and attachment patterns. These formative early months of motherhood can be a time of significant foment, evoking reflections on past and present attachment relationships precipitating surprising and strong affective responses to "ghosts" from the past [30] as well as more positive "angels" [31]. Being a new experience, the mother's thoughts and feelings towards her newborn baby and her new caring role are less established and likely to be more flexible. The mother's patterns of behaviour are still in formation and responses are not yet predictable and anticipated, allowing opportunity for flexibility and change. Consequently, the MBN program is offered within the first six months post birth to seize this opportunity of flexibility in the mother-infant dyad.

3.2 Infant as participant

From birth, the infant has capacity for primary intersubjectivity; to be engaged as a person in their own right [32, 33]. More so, the infant's subjective sense of self is actually dependent on the quality of the interactions with those they relate to [33]. Engaging the mother in isolation misses an opportunity to directly contribute to the infant's development, the quality of the mother-infant interactions and the promotion of infant mental health [34]. Paradoxically due to neuroplasticity, the vulnerable infant is the most receptive and adaptive member in the dyad, making them a potent agent of change in the relationship. Stirred by the enlivened infant, the mother's attachment systems can be activated, creating opportunity for reorganisation of internal representations, role and emerging attachment patterns [26], as well as inhibiting disorganised attachment in infants [35].

During the MBN group, facilitators express curiosity and interest in the infant's experience, marking moments of brief exchange with curiosity and delight, which serve to legitimise the infant's experience. This sensitive and responsive exchange over time, supports the infant's developing sense of self and capacity to regulate emotions [36]. For example, while holding the infant's gaze and providing marked mirroring of the baby's expression the facilitator may say, "I wonder what you might be feeling as your mother shared that story? I think it makes your mummy feel sad; does it make you feel sad too?" The embodied act responding to the infant and holding him in mind as a thinking, feeling being is a central aspect of MBN. Such interventions support the mother's capacity for perspective-taking, beyond her own experience and adult concerns, to consider the perspective and experience of her infant [37].

As we (facilitator, mother, and group) practice holding a reflective stance, wondering aloud about the baby's efforts and shared moments of meeting, we consider how the infant's external behaviour is informed by his internal experiences. We acknowledge times when the infant and mother share joyful moments, as well as acknowledge (without judgement) shared moments of uncomfortable affect. The infant serves as the 'honest' member of the dyad, enacting feelings that are shared but not necessarily expressed by the mother [38, 39].

Infant-focused moments occur spontaneously, as well as formally through a weekly group practice derived from the Irish Gaelic definition of curiosity, ábhar le ionadh, which translates "to watch with wonder" [40]. Mothers quietly watch their baby, invited to wonder about what the infant may be experiencing, reflecting on their possible thoughts, feelings, urges and bodily sensations. The curious, 'not-knowing' stance is both an important marker of all mentalizing interventions and core component in the child-led psychotherapeutic program, Watch Wait and Wonder [41]. Exercising a state of presence and attention with the infant is especially powerful for mothers that may ordinarily withdraw (absorbed in their own internal world) or for the mother preoccupied with their infant's externalised behaviour (feeding, sleeping, or crying). It may also bring intrusive patterns of attachment behaviour to light, that are observed and held in mind by the facilitator. Reflecting on 'in-the-moment' experiences can illuminate past narratives and distortions that inform the mother's internal working model, shaping the way she responds to her infant [42]. It can offer a window into the mother's activated internal world that, if the infant were not present, may have taken longer or remained hidden from sight.

3.3 The group as a containing space

The MBN facilitators seek to provide a supportive relationship for the mother and the babies much like the role of a mother for an infant; described by Winnicott [5] as a necessary "holding" and Bion [43] as "containing". Scaffolded by agreed group guidelines and processes, the group can form a kind, non-judgemental space for the mother and infant to express distress, anxiety, and pain. Once expressed, these projections can be returned in a modified and palatable form [44]. The group provides a safe container from which its members (mothers and infants) can begin to trust in the observations and feedback made by other members and become more receptive to new learnings. The experience of authenticity and openness can support the mother to develop an experiential understanding of social environments and interactions, a process defined as epistemic trust [24]. The benefits of epistemic trust are expected to continue well after the facilitated group ends, leading to sustained supportive relationships between group members, which act as a steppingstone to wider social contexts.

The role of the MBN facilitators is to hold both the mother and the infant in mind as thinking, feeling beings whose experiences and behaviours are meaningful. The facilitators scaffold the dyads experience, noticing strengths in both infant and mother, creating opportunities for brief attuned interactions to be acknowledged and amplified. The role of the group then, is to offer the infant enlivening experiences that will support his engagement with others, in his exploration as well as providing an emotionally containing presence when the infant is seeking support to regulate emotions. The facilitators are also offered containment from their regular supervision, which completes a nested set of relationships much like a babushka doll, one contained within the next: supervisor, facilitators, mother and infant (A similar 'Containment Model' is presented in [45]).

The group process acts as a holding environment for the vulnerable mother [46] as facilitators carefully narrate changes and absences in the group, including preparation for the eventual group closure, as thoughts of separation can activate strong feelings [23]. When disruptions are repaired, it helps inform the members by providing suggested scripts on how minor family ruptures and repairs can be managed within trust relationships. When a member of the group shares an affective state, the containing experience of marked mirroring can be amplified and nuanced as the multiple members provide a "hall of mirrors" response that offers differing affective intensity and hues [47]. The group can also offer some distance when a member listens to another's experience, she can gain insight into aspects of her own internal world that may have been previously obscured. The process of identifying one's own experience within the story of another member is both validating as well as normalising, alleviating feelings of isolation and shame. Establishing the service within the community instead of hospital setting, also helps destigmatise their experience.

3.4 Enhancing mentalizing

Mentalizing is a concept that has origins in psychodynamic theory, attachment theory and cognitive psychology [5, 43, 48–50]. The concept of parental mentalizing provides a well-established theory and mode of relationship-focused intervention (Mentalization-Based Treatment) that is accessible across disciplines [51–54]. Evidence suggests that parental mentalizing is a central process in the intergenerational transmission of attachment patterns [55, 56], with poor parental mentalizing predictive of children's insecure [57] and disorganised attachment [58]. The way a mother cares for her infant is informed by her own experience of being parented, explicitly in behaviours, and implicitly through enacting her internal working model [30]. A recent study of these processes [59] found that mothers' poor mentalizing of their own early attachment relationships was predictive of negative parenting behaviours, which were strongly related to attachment insecurity and disorganisation. Interestingly, promoting maternal sensitivity behaviours alone (via psychoeducation) has not been found to mitigate the transmission of the caregiver's adult attachment patterns to the infant [60].

Time in each session is dedicated to supporting mother-infant play and experiencing or 'being-with' the emotions and mental states of the infant. Conversations are facilitated so mothers reflect on attachment relationships - both representations from her childhood and her current perceptions of her baby. Through facial expressions, gestures, talking or vocalising, and actions (including play), a mother can support her infant to recognise his own internal state and regulate his emotions. It is through experiencing a mother's mentalizing that a child can 'make sense' of his environment, supporting him to develop affect regulation, mitigating against stress arousal, and promoting the development of secure patterns of attachment and sense of personal agency [61, 62]. This engagement also contributes to the develop his sense of subjective self [63]. The MBN facilitator thinks about and relates to the mothers and babies as thinking, feeling beings. Through repetition, modelling curiosity about internal states is transmitted to the mothers, encouraging them to consider their own and their infants' internal states.

This curiosity and openness in thinking helps to develop the skill of metacognition, so rather than being 'in it' the mother is able to think 'on it' which enables her to examine her internal working model and how she views the intentions of her child and her own self [60]. Through practicing this type of perspective taking, the mother's mentalizing capacity is stretched and strengthened. This way of being, once nurtured in the group can continue to develop beyond the life of the group and is passed forward through the infant-parent relationship.

4. Outcomes

4.1 Intended outcomes for the mother

As the mother seeks to care for her infant, the facilitators may notice that the mother expresses strong emotions, ambivalent or negative feelings in what she says about her infant or in the way she responds or handles him. The facilitators emotionally contain the expressed state, allowing the mother to talk about her experiences, without fear of abandonment, intrusion, or criticism. A mother who is able to articulate her longing, or to mourn her loss or express her anger or despair within the context of a nurturing relationship may become clearer about her relational history and more emotionally available and sensitive to her infant [30, 64, 65]. In the safety of the supportive relationship, the mother may become more able to mentalize emotionally charged events and this lowers her epistemic vigilance [24]. This capacity will supports her to revisit the difficult experience in a more resourceful way, giving her opportunity to better understand and integrate the feelings that threaten the developing attachment relationship [24, 30]. Well-regulated affect between the dyad can be internalised into the child's developing internal working model and 'secure base' attachment relationship [66], reducing the risk of intergenerational transmission [57, 67]. The mother learns how to provide contingent responses to the infant, so the infant can register his mental states as a coherent part of himself, rather than as random or alien [68]. This learning is possibly through the development of epistemic trust [24] and is then applied in everyday life. Based on these principles and understandings, the outcomes of MBN for the mother are summarised in **Figure 1**.

4.2 Intended outcomes for the infant

The infants developing sense of subjective self, as a separate entity from the caregiver, is a central organising process of psychological development [63, 69]. The group provides a transitional space for the infant [70], where he can observe those around him, noticing similarities and differences, and feel safe enough to explore new experiences of self. This can be a powerful learning opportunity especially for a socially isolated mother and baby, as it offers a space in which alternate expressions of thinking and feeling can be experienced and offered [37].

Ways of being together become imbedded in the infant's procedural memory, forming an internal representation of how others relate to him and how he relates to others. These repeated "serve and return" experiences between the infant and others, most especially their caregivers, form the infant's internal working model [66]. Although able to be revised and elaborated on, the internal working model is largely established early in infancy and acts to inform future ways of relating [71]. The emotionally containing and contingent interactions of the group support the infant to foster their developing subjective self, sense of agency, and capacity for emotional regulation and secure attachment (see **Figure 1**).

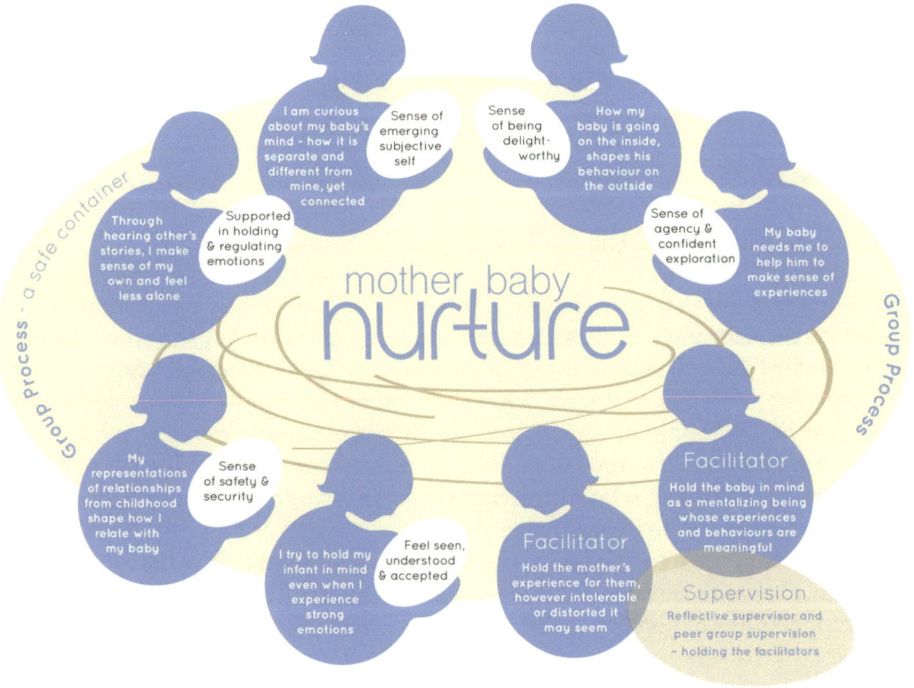

Figure 1.
Mother-Baby Nurture outcomes model.

5. Conclusion

We have outlined four key aspects of the Mother-Baby Nurture group program. Firstly, the early parent-infant relationship is understood as central in supporting better health and developmental outcomes for the developing child. Then we described how the infant is welcomed and included as a participant in the group, using moments of interaction as material for shared pleasure and reflective discussion. Within the safe environment of the group, the mothers are able to reflect on their relationships present and past, allowing distress and distortions to become seen and contained. Finally, the facilitators model a mentalizing stance of curiosity, supporting the mother to reflect on feelings and longings, as well as considering the experiences of her baby and other group participants.

This program offers a therapeutic experience for vulnerable families. Prioritising the infant-parent attachment relationship in tertiary services can prove difficult where treatment of acute maternal psychopathology can overshadow the experience of the infant. Mother-Baby Nurture delivers a unique targeted service for vulnerable families during a critical window in the infant's development while the tender caregiver relationship is in formation. This relationship-focused program can be delivered by infant mental health clinicians from all disciplines. It gives a family an experience that can foster a sense of trust, providing a stepping-stone to other protective support services, as well as engagement with the community at large.

Acknowledgements

The authors express gratitude to the infants and their mothers' who inform and inspire this program and who were willing to watch with wonder with us. Thank you to the Mother-Baby Nurture facilitators and supervisors whose reflections continue to shape the program and the brave pioneers that piloted the first group more than ten years ago.

Author details

Sharon Cooke[1], Dawson Cooke[2*] and Sue Coleson[1]

1 Playgroup WA, Perth, Australia

2 Curtin University, Perth, Australia

*Address all correspondence to: dawson.cooke@curtin.edu.au

References

[1] Shonkoff JP, Phillips DA. From Neurons to Neighbourhoods: The Science of Early Childhood Development. Washington, D.C: National Academy Press; 2000

[2] Parsons CE, Young KS, Murray L, Stein A, Kringelbach M. The functional neuroanatomy of the evolving parent–infant relationship. Progress in Neurobiology. 2010;**91**(3):220-241

[3] Lyons-Ruth K, Todd Manly J, Von Klitzing K, Tamminen T, Emde R, Fitzgerald H, et al. The worldwide burden of infant mental and emotional disorder: Report of the task force of the world association for infant mental health. Infant Mental Health Journal. 2017;**38**(6):695-705

[4] Assink M, Spruit A, Schuts M, Lindauer R, van der Put CE, Stams G-JJ. The intergenerational transmission of child maltreatment: A three-level meta-analysis. Child Abuse & Neglect. 2018;**84**:131-145

[5] Winnicott DW. The theory of the parent-infant relationship. International Journal of Psycho-Analysis. 1960;**41**:585-595

[6] Bowlby J. A Secure Base: Parent-Child Attachment and Healthy Human Development. London: Routledge; 1988

[7] Sharp C, Fonagy P. The parent's capacity to treat the child as a psychological agent: Constructs, measures and implications for developmental psychopathology. Social Development. 2008;**17**(3):737-754

[8] Fonagy P, Target M. Attachment and reflective function: Their role in self-organization. Development and Psychopathology. 1997;**9**:21

[9] Zeanah CH, Lieberman A. Relationship-specific disorder of early childhood. In: Zeanah CH, editor. Handbook of Infant Mental Health. 4th ed. New York: Guilford Press; 2019. pp. 467-483

[10] Cowan PA, Cowan CP. Attachment theory: Seven unresolved issues and questions for future research. Research in Human Development. 2007;**4**(3-4):181-201

[11] Grossmann K, Grossmann KE, Kindler H. Early care and the roots of attachment and partnership representations: The Bielefeld and Regensburg longitudinal studies. In: Grossmann K, Grossmann KE, Waters E, editors. Attachment from Infancy to Adulthood: The Major Longitudinal Studies. New York: Guildford Press; 2005. pp. 98-136

[12] Osofsky JD, Thomas K. What is infant mental health? Zero to Three. 2012;**33**(2):9

[13] Sleed M, Li E, Vainieri I, Midgley N. The Evidence Base for Psychoanalytic and Psychodynamic Interventions with Children under 5 Years of Age and their Caregivers: A Systematic Review and Meta-Analysis. London: The Anna Freud Centre; 2022

[14] Cooke S, Cooke D, Coleson S. Mother-Baby Nurture Facilitation Manual. 2019

[15] Cooke S, Cooke DC, Hauck Y. Relationship focused mother–infant groups: Preliminary evaluation of improvements in maternal mental health, parenting confidence, and

parental reflective functioning. Infant Mental Health Journal. 2023:1-15. DOI: 10.1002/imhj.22080

[16] Ippen CG, Norona CR, Thomas K. From tenet to practice: Putting diversity-informed services into action. Zero to Three. 2012;**33**(2):23-28

[17] McHale J, Phares V. From dyads to family systems: A bold new direction for infant mental health practice. Zero to Three Journal. 2015;**35**(5):2-10

[18] Panter-Brick C, Burgess A, Eggerman M, McAllister F, Pruett K, Leckman JF. Practitioner review: Engaging fathers – Recommendations for a game change in parenting interventions based on a systematic review of the global evidence. Journal of Child Psychology and Psychiatry. 2014;**55**(11):1187-1212

[19] Tomlin AM, Weatherston DJ, Pavkov T. Critical components of reflective supervision: Responses from expert supervisors in the field. Infant Mental Health Journal. 2014;**35**(1):70-80

[20] Weatherston D, Weigand RF, Weigand B. Reflective supervision: Supporting reflection as a cornerstone for competency. Zero to Three. 2010;**31**(2):22-30

[21] Weatherston D, Barron C. What does a reflective supervisory relationship look like? In: Heller SS, Gilkerson L, editors. A Practical Guide to Reflective Supervision. Washington, D.C: Zero to Three Press; 2009. pp. 63-82

[22] Pawl J. The therapeutic relationship as human connectedness: Being held in another's mind. Zero to Three. 1995;**15**(4):1-5

[23] James J. Parent-infant psychotherapy in groups. In: Baradon T, Biseo M, Broughton C, James J, Joyce A, editors. The Practice of Psychoanalytic Parent-Infant Psychotherapy: Claiming the Baby. New York: Routledge; 2016. pp. 138-157

[24] Fonagy P, Campbell C, Bateman A. Mentalizing, attachment, and epistemic trust in group therapy. International Journal of Group Psychotherapy. 2017;**67**(2):176-201

[25] Kalland M, Fagerlund Å, von Koskull M, Pajulo M. Families first: The development of a new mentalization-based group intervention for first-time parents to promote child development and family health. Primary Health Care Research & Development. 2016;**17**(1):3-17

[26] Stern DN. The motherhood constellation. A unified view of parent-infant psychotherapy. 1995

[27] Heim C, Owens MJ, Plotsky PM, Nemeroff CB. Persistent changes in corticotropin-releasing factor systems due to early life stress: Relationship to the pathophysiology of major depression and post-traumatic stress disorder. Psychopharmacology Bulletin. 1997;**33**(2):185

[28] Lyons-Ruth K. The interface between attachment and intersubjectivity: Perspective from the longitudinal study of disorganized attachment. Psychoanalytic Inquiry. 2006;**26**(4):595-616

[29] Groh AM, Fearon RP, van IjzendoornMH,Bakermans-KranenburgMJ, Roisman GI. Attachment in the early life course: Meta-analytic evidence for its role in socioemotional development. Child Development Perspectives. 2017;**11**(1):70-76

[30] Fraiberg S, Adelson E, Shapiro V. Ghosts in the nursery: A psychoanalytic

approach to the problems of impaired infant-mother relationships. Journal of the American Academy of Child Psychiatry. 1975;**14**(3):387-421

[31] Lieberman AF, Padron E, Van Horn P, Harris WW. Angels in the nursery: The intergenerational transmission of benevolent parental influences. Infant Mental Health Journal. 2005;**26**(6):504-520

[32] Trevarthen C, Aitken KJ. Infant intersubjectivity: Research, theory, and clinical applications. Journal of Child Psychology and Psychiatry. 2001;**42**(1):3-48

[33] Shai D, Belsky J. When words just won't do: Introducing parental embodied mentalizing. Child Development Perspectives. 2011;**5**(3):173-180

[34] Zeanah CH. Handbook of Infant Mental Health. 4th ed. New York: Guildford Press; 2018

[35] Facompré CR, Bernard K, Waters TE. Effectiveness of interventions in preventing disorganized attachment: A meta-analysis. Development and Psychopathology. 2018;**30**(1):1-11

[36] Thomson-Salo F. Engaging with the baby as a person: Early intervention with parents and infants. In: Paul C, Thomson-Salo F, editors. The Baby as Subject: Clinical Studies in Infant-Parent Therapy. London: Karnac Books; 2013. pp. 7-16

[37] Joyce A. The parent–infant relationship and infant mental health. In: Baradon T, Biseo M, Broughton C, James J, Joyce A, editors. The Practice of Psychoanalytic Parent-Infant Psychotherapy: Claiming the Baby. New York: Routledge; 2016. pp. 29-53

[38] Morgan A. What I am trying to do when I see an infant with his or her parents. In: Paul C, Thomson-Salo F, editors. The Baby as Subject: Clinical Studies in Infant-Parent Therapy. London: Karnac Books; 2013. pp. 1-6

[39] Paul C, Thomson-Salo F. The Baby as Subject: Clinical Studies in Infant-Parent Therapy. Karnac Books; 2013

[40] Ó Tuama P. To Watch with Wonder. Personal correspondence with author 2017

[41] Cohen NJ, Muir E, Lojkasek M, Muir R, Parker CJ, Barwick M, et al. Watch, wait, and wonder: Testing the effectiveness of a new approach to mother-infant psychotherapy. Infant Mental Health Journal. 1999;**20**(4):429-451

[42] Onions C. The ordinary devoted group: Developing a parent and baby psychotherapy group. In: Celebi M, editor. Weaving the Cradle: Facilitating Groups to Promote Attunement and Bonding between Parents, their Babies and Toddlers. London: Singing Dragon; 2017. pp. 106-119

[43] Bion WR. A theory of thinking. The International journal of Psycho-analysis. 1962;**43**:306

[44] Baradon T, Joyce A. The theory of psychoanalytic parent-infant psychotherapy. In: Baradon T, Biseo M, Broughton C, James J, Joyce A, editors. The Practice of Psychoanalytic Parent-Infant Psychotherapy: Claiming the Baby. East Sussex: Routledge; 2016. pp. 25-40

[45] Underdown A. Baby steps: A relationship-based perinatal group programme. In: Celebi M, editor. Weaving the Cradle: Facilitating Groups to Promote Attunement and Bonding between Parents, their Babies and Toddlers. London: Singing Dragon; 2017. pp. 156-167

[46] Grienenberger J. Group process as a holding environment facilitating the development of the parental reflective function: Commentary on the article by arietta Slade. Psychoanalytic Inquiry. 2006;**26**(4):668-675

[47] Weinberg H, Toder M. The hall of mirrors in small, large and virtual groups. Group Analysis. 2004;**37**(4):492-507

[48] Main M, Kaplan N, Cassidy J. Security in infancy, childhood, and adulthood: A move to the level of representation. Monographs of the Society for Research in Child Development. 1985;**50**(1/2):66-104

[49] Goldman AI. Theory of mind. In: The Oxford Handbook of Philosophy of Cognitive Science. New York: University Oxford Press; 2012. pp. 402-424

[50] Fonagy P. Attachment Theory and Psychoanalysis. London: Karnac; 2001

[51] Slade A. Reflective parenting programs: Theory and development. Psychoanalytic Inquiry. 2006;**26**(4):640-647

[52] Bateman A, Fonagy P. Mentalization-based treatment. Psychoanalytic Inquiry. 2013;**33**(6):595-613

[53] Katznelson H. Reflective functioning: A review. Clinical Psychology Review. 2014;**34**(2):107-117

[54] Malda-Castillo J, Browne C, Perez-Algorta G. Mentalization-based treatment and its evidence-base status: A systematic literature review. Psychology and Psychotherapy: Theory, Research and Practice. 2018;**92**(4):465-498

[55] Fonagy P, Target M. Bridging the transmission gap: An end to an important mystery of attachment research? Attachment and Human Development. 2005;**7**(3):333-343

[56] Bernier A, Dozier M. Bridging the attachment transmission gap: The role of maternal mind-mindedness. International Journal of Behavioral Development. 2003;**27**(4):355-365

[57] Slade A, Grienenberger J, Bernbach E, Levy D, Locker A. Maternal reflective functioning, attachment, and the transmission gap: A preliminary study. Attachment and Human Development. 2005;**7**(3):283-298

[58] Grienenberger J, Kelly K, Slade A. Maternal reflective functioning, mother-infant affective communication, and infant attachment: Exploring the link between mental states and observed caregiving behaviour in the intergenerational transmission of attachment. Attachment and Human Development. 2005;**7**(3):299-311

[59] Ensink K, Normandin L, Plamondon A, Berthelot N, Fonagy P. Intergenerational pathways from reflective functioning to infant attachment through parenting. Canadian Journal of Behavioural Science/ Revue canadienne des sciences du comportement. 2016;**48**(1):9-18

[60] Grienenberger J, Denham W, Reynolds D. Reflective and mindful parenting: A new relational model of assessment, prevention, and early intervention. In: Luyten P, Mayes LC, Fonagy P, Target M, Blatt SJ, editors. Handbook of Psychodynamic Approaches to Psychopathology. New York: Guildord Press; 2015

[61] Slade A. Parental reflective functioning: An introduction. Attachment and Human Development. 2005;**7**:269-281

[62] Ensink K, Mayes L. The development of Mentalisation in children from a theory of mind

perspective. Psychoanalytic Inquiry. 2010;**30**(4):301-337

[63] Fonagy P, Gergely G, Target M. The parent-infant dyad and the construction of the subjective self. Journal of Child Psychology and Psychiatry. 2007;**48**(3-4):288-328

[64] Stinson S, Tableman B, Weatherston D. Guidelines for Infant Mental Health Practice. East Lansing: Michigan Association for Infant Mental Health; 2000

[65] Schore JR, Schore AN. Modern attachment theory: The central role of affect regulation in development and treatment. Clinical Social Work Journal. 2008;**36**(1):9-20

[66] Bowlby J. Attachment and Loss: Attachment. London: Hogarth Press; 1969

[67] Allen JG, Fonagy P, editors. Handbook of Mentalization-Based Treatment. West Sussex: John Wiley & Sons; 2006

[68] Berthelot N, Ensink K, Bernazzani O, Normandin L, Luyten P, Fonagy P. Intergenerational transmission of attachment in abused and neglected mothers: The role of trauma-specific reflective functioning. Infant Mental Health Journal. 2015;**36**(2):200-212

[69] Stern DN. The Interpersonal World of the Infant: A View from Psychoanalysis and Developmental Psychology. New York: Karnac Books; 1985

[70] Winnicott DW. Playing and Reality. London: Travistock Publications; 1971

[71] Sherman LJ, Rice K, Cassidy J. Infant capacities related to building internal working models of attachment figures: A theoretical and empirical review. Developmental Review. 2015;**37**:109-141

Chapter 6

As New Challenges Emerge, Africa is Still Faced with Sociocultural and Health System Challenges Leading to Maternal Mortality

Thendo Gertie Makhado, Lufuno Makhado, Mutshinyalo Lizzy Netshikeweta and Azwidihwi Rose Tshililo

Abstract

Globally, the most crucial element of development strategies is a decrease in maternal mortality. Every 2 minutes, a pregnant woman dies from complications related to pregnancy or childbirth. According to studies, the majority of pregnancy and delivery difficulties are mostly influenced by sociocultural and health system factors. PUBMED, Google Scholar, National EDT, EBSCOHost, and Science Direct databases were used to find relevant articles. The process for choosing relevant and qualified articles was based on a PRISMA flowchart. The standard of the accepted articles was evaluated using the Critical Appraisal Skill Program (CASP) checklists. This study employed a thematic analysis, and in the articles on sociocultural and healthcare system factors influencing maternal mortality, six themes and 23 sub-themes were found. It was determined that most women choose to consult traditional experts during pregnancy or childbirth rather than health facilities, and that there is little interaction between societal expectations and the healthcare system, which further contributes to problems and maternal mortality. This study found that social, cultural, and health system factors may directly and indirectly contribute to maternal mortality. It is also recommended that cultural norms and health system norms collaborate together to reduce maternal mortality.

Keywords: maternal mortality, sociocultural factors, health system factors, pregnancy, childbirth

1. Introduction

A worldwide crisis has been identified: maternal mortality. Despite all the efforts put in place, maternal mortality has been reported by the World Health Organization (WHO) [1] to be high in African countries. Despite various methods and estimates, it is a fact that Nigeria has the highest maternal mortality rate in Africa. The rate is considerably higher than the global average of 290 maternal deaths per 100,000

IntechOpen

live births [2–4]. Sub-Saharan Africa continues to have the highest rates of maternal mortality in the entire world. Up to half of all maternal deaths worldwide caused by pregnancy-related complications occur in sub-Saharan Africa [5–7]. According to the literature, sub-Saharan Africa has the highest maternal death rate in the world [8]. Moreover, Mozambique is one of the sub-Saharan African nations with a high death rate of 500 per 100,000 live births [8–11]. Maternal mortality is more prevalent in poor households than in rich households in sub-Saharan countries, according to studies comparing maternal mortality between rich and poor households [12–15]. This is mainly because poor households lack the resources to pay for quality prenatal and postpartum care. Although maternal mortality in South Africa has decreased compared to other African nations, it is still above the objective. The WHO [1] underlined this objective, noting that it aimed to "reduce the global maternal mortality rate (MMR) to fewer than 70 per 100,000 births, with no nation having a maternal mortality rate that is more than twice the global average." Maternal mortality has decreased in South Africa, according to Moodley et al. [16]. The number of deaths resulting from specific conditions that increase maternal mortality is still stubbornly high. Much research has been carried out to determine the causes of maternal mortality in several African nations, including South Africa [2, 16–18]. However, maternal mortality is still increasing [1, 19]. Cardiovascular problems, obstetric hemorrhage, eclampsia, and ectopic pregnancy are factors in maternal mortality that have been extensively studied [20, 21]. According to a study conducted in Africa, traditional practices and health system factors may cause pregnant women to wait longer before seeking medical attention, which increases the risk of maternal mortality [22–24]. This indicates that there are some cultural beliefs and health system factors that may increase the risk of maternal mortality.

This systematic review seeks to present a clear or comprehensive picture of sociocultural practices/contributors and aspects of the health system that have been identified as factors influencing maternal mortality, specifically in scholarly papers of studies conducted in Africa. It appears that no systematic review of the expanding body of knowledge on this subject, specifically in Africa, has been published. Consequently, the researcher conducted a methodical examination of the available data on sociocultural practices and healthcare system factors that play a role in maternal mortality in Africa, and pinpointed the elements that were referenced in the studies mentioned earlier. The review question was, "What are the sociocultural and health systems factors contributing to maternal mortality in Africa?"

2. Methods and materials

The aim of this systematic review was to identify the sociocultural and health system factors influencing maternal mortality in Africa. The review utilized specific search strategies, inclusion criteria, study selection, data abstraction, and article evaluation methods. The search was conducted using various databases including PUBMED, Google Scholar, National EDT, EBSCOHost, and Science Direct, and the search terms used were "sociocultural factors," "health system factors," "traditional practices," "contribut*," "maternal mortality," and "Africa." The inclusion criteria involved articles published in English, between 2012 and 2022, conducted on humans, using both qualitative and quantitative methods, and focusing on sociocultural and health system factors contributing to maternal mortality in Africa. Participants included pregnant women or those who had given birth within 42 days. The PRISMA flow diagram [25] was used to select relevant studies and eliminate duplicates. All articles were initially screened using their titles and abstracts; they included PubMed (n = 24), EBSCOHOST (n = 227), National EDT (n = 129), ScienceDirect (n = 1922), and Google Scholar (n = 18,401), for a total of 20,703. Additionally, 2666 duplicates were eliminated from the list, leaving a total of 180,367. Following a review of the themes and abstracts of the studies, 7633 studies were eliminated. Of the 10,404 studies that met the inclusion criteria—which included being published in English and being located on the African continent and having a publication year between 2012 and 2022—2110,383 studies were excluded (see PRISMA Flowchart in **Figure 1**). After screening and eliminating articles that did not meet the inclusion criteria, eight articles matched the criteria. Permission was not required since all articles were publicly available.

The researcher conducted a comparison of collected data and extracted information. They gathered information on all research articles and literature reviews that met the inclusion criteria, including the study's author, publication year, location, aims, population, outcomes, and limitations. More details on the study's characteristics that were examined during the review are available in **Table 1**. (Refer to **Table 1** for further information.)

Quality assessment only applied to the entire texts of the papers that were selected and met the criteria for inclusion (see **Table 2**). Utilizing Critical Appraisal Skill Program (CASP), all the researches included in the review were methodically and

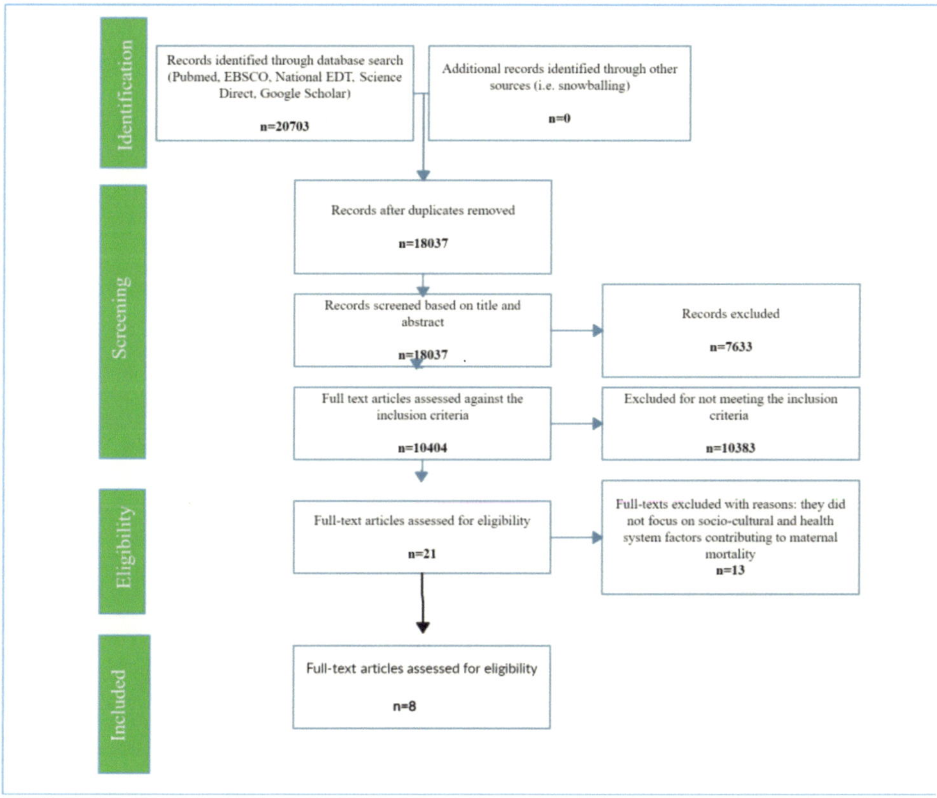

Figure 1.
Study selection procedure (PRISMA flowchart).

Author and year	Country	Objectives of the article	Study design	Population	Documented outcomes	Limitations
Kea et al. [26]	Ethiopia	The aim of this study was to identify the factors that influence the frequency of maternal health service utilization at the primary healthcare unit (PHCU) level among rural populations in the Sidama zone, south Ethiopia. Additionally, the study aimed to develop strategies for improving the quality of maternal health services.	Explorative qualitative study	The population for this study included community members such as women, men, traditional birth attendants (TBAs), and local kebele administrators, as well as health professionals and health extension workers.	This study's findings revealed that various factors affect access to high-quality treatment, including traditional and cultural beliefs, distance to medical facilities, previous successful deliveries, and trust in TBAs.	Due to the recent prohibition of TBAs from conducting delivery services, they were often hesitant to provide detailed information.
Bucher et al. [27]	Kenya	The aim of the study was to understand the practices and protocols adopted by traditional birth attendants within our catchment area and to provide valuable insights into the discussion surrounding their roles.	Descriptive study	Traditional birth attendants (TBAs)	The results of the study showed a positive association between traditional birth attendants (TBAs) and healthcare facilities. In addition, harmful practices that can lead to maternal mortality were identified.	The conclusions of this study were drawn from self-reported data. This descriptive study focused on a limited sample of traditional birth attendants from Western Kenya, so the findings may not be entirely representative of TBAs in other regions of Kenya or in other countries.
Berhan & Berhan [28]	Ethiopia	To make a rough estimate of the impact of various socioeconomic and cultural factors on maternal mortality.	Literature review	The study population consisted of electronic databases from Ethiopian Central Statistics Agency, MEASURE DHS, World Health Organization, and PUBMED.	The study identified low contraceptive utilization, risky traditional practices, low economic status, and poor adult literacy rates as key factors that contribute to Ethiopia's persistently high rates of maternal and perinatal mortality.	

Author and year	Country	Objectives of the article	Study design	Population	Documented outcomes	Limitations
Abubakar; Yohanna & Zubairu [29]	Nigeria	The study aimed to explore the impact of cultural beliefs and values on obstetric complications experienced by women who delivered their babies at Yusuf Dantsoho Memorial Hospital in Tudun Wada, Kaduna.	Cross-sectional quantitative study	The study population was comprised of women who delivered babies at Yusuf Dantsoho Memorial Hospital in Tudun Wada, Kaduna during April 2014.	The results of the research align with the universal report on common obstetric issues. Nevertheless, other cultural factors were making the situation more complex by preventing women from seeking medical care.	
Sibiya et al. [30]	South Africa	The aim was to explore the factors that impacted the access of pregnant women from the rural community of KwaMkhizwana to antenatal care (ANC) services. This research sought to investigate the variables that affected the utilization of antenatal care (ANC) services by pregnant women living in the rural community of KwaMkhizwana.	The qualitative study employed an exploratory descriptive, and contextual research design	The study population consisted of pregnant women residing in the remote area and all nursing specialties employed at the three healthcare facilities.	Most of the pregnant women who participated in the study reported experiencing restricted availability to healthcare services.	The study involved pregnant women who were 18 years old and above. However, some pregnant women were unable to participate because they did not use the accessible healthcare facilities in the region.
Muhwava, Morojele & London [31]	South Africa	The objective was to explore the correlation between psychosocial factors and the prompt initiation of antenatal care (ANC) and appropriate attendance frequency of ANC visits among women in South Africa.	Cross-sectional quantitative research design	The research focused solely on women who had experienced pregnancy and were therefore eligible to participate in the study.	The study found no noteworthy correlations between psychosocial factors and appropriate ANC attendance frequency in the urban location.	The utilization of an existing dataset restricted the research to utilizing the survey questionnaire design for data gathering purposes.

Author and year	Country	Objectives of the article	Study design	Population	Documented outcomes	Limitations
Marchie [32]	Nigeria	The aim was to investigate the sociocultural factors that impact maternal mortality in the Edo South Senatorial District..	The research employed a descriptive survey methodology.	The study population comprised of all married females of reproductive age, healthcare workers, and relatives of women who passed away during pregnancy, childbirth, or the postpartum period.	According to the study findings, cultural and traditional factors were found to potentially heighten the chances of maternal mortality. Additionally, harmful traditional practices like female genital mutilation were identified as sociocultural factors that contribute to maternal mortality.	
Ansong et al. [33]	Southern Ghana	The purpose of this study was to examine the impact of beliefs and practices on maternal and child healthcare services.	The research utilized both narrative and phenomenology study methodologies.	The study involved individuals from the community, including pregnant women and women with children under the age of five.	The study results indicated that sociocultural beliefs and practices were present during the prenatal, delivery, and postnatal stages. These behaviors were found to be both positive and negative. The tradition of seclusion and the delayed initiation of antenatal care was seen as a means of protecting the pregnancy from evil forces. The study also noted that women who take herbal medications to hasten labor tended to prefer home deliveries with the aid of traditional birth attendants.	

Table 1.
Characteristics of the selected studies.

Authors and year	Study design	Assessment of Studies
Marchie [32]	Descriptive survey method	80%
Muhwava et al. [31]	Cross-sectional quantitative method	70%
Sibiya et al. [30]	Qualitative, exploratory, descriptive design	69%
Berhan & Berhan [28]	Literature review	60%
Bucher et al. [27]	Descriptive study	85%
Kea et al. [26]	Explorative qualitative study	90%
Abubakar et al. [29]	Cross-sectional quantitative study	70%
Ansong et al. [33]	Qualitative, both narrative and phenomenology study designs	80%

Table 2.
Appraisal of studies using CASP.

meticulously assessed to determine their value, applicability, and credibility. The included studies' overall quality ranged from 60 to 90%, with an average of 75% exhibiting moderate to high quality.

A thematic analysis was performed to identify similar patterns among the articles reviewed. The similar patterns were grouped together, forming themes, and the following were the themes that emerged from the review: community members' opinions about the state of maternal health (n = 8), culture-related factors (n = 7), ppregnant-women-related factors (n = 4), healthcare system factors (n = 4), choice of care (n = 5), and Traditional birth attendant (TBA)-related factors (n = 2).

3. Results

According to the studies examined in this review, the majority of women prefer TBAs over medical visits, despite the fact that doing so carries a significant risk of complications that could result in maternal mortality. This showed that women's decisions about their healthcare are influenced by a variety of other factors. Six themes and 23 subthemes emerged regarding sociocultural and health system factors/practices contributing to maternal mortality from the included articles (see **Table 3**). The themes that emerged included culture-related factors, pregnant-women-related factors, health system factors, choice of care, and traditional-birth-attendant-related factors.

3.1 Community members' opinions about the state of maternal health

The reviewed studies have shown that a variety of factors, including ignorance (n = 7, 100%), traditional birth attendance experience (n = 3, 43%), prior child-birth experience (n = 3, 43%), perceptions of risk (n = 1, 14%), and facility-based experiences (n = 2, 29%), affect people's perceptions of maternal health [26–32]. Lack of knowledge was revealed to be the main factor influencing how community members perceive maternal mortality. According to Meh et al. [4], Batist [5], Yemane & Tiruneh [6], Ahinkorah et al. [7], Central Intelligence Agency [8], Buor & Bream [9], and Adde et al. [10], the lack of awareness about risk factors and problems may contribute to maternal mortality, which may result in most women delaying booking for antenatal care (ANC) and opting to deliver their babies in hospitals rather than at home. Lack of information has been identified as the primary barrier to receiving maternal health services in a study by Kea et al. [26], and the majority of women who have delivered at home say they would not do so if they were aware of the advantages of receiving maternal health services in health facilities.

Through the reviewed studies, most women's perceptions regarding maternal health have been reported to be affected by their previous experiences during pregnancy, their perceptions regarding the risks associated with maternal mortality, and their earlier experiences with the healthcare facilities' services during childbirth [26, 27, 31]. According to Kea et al. [26], some women who experienced issues during delivery at the healthcare facilities and were passionately assisted may not think twice about going to the facilities during their pregnancy, childbirth, and recovery time. However, other women had unpleasant experiences with prior deliveries in medical facilities due to issues in the healthcare system, such as the unfavorable attitudes of medical staff, the facilities' remote locations, and a lack of privacy, which led them to choose home birth to medical facilities. Culture-influenced lack of decision-making on the part of women regarding their past pregnancies is another element influencing how people view maternal health. According to research by Kea et al. [26] and Marchie [32], women are never given the opportunity to make decisions throughout pregnancy, childbirth, or following delivery. Yet, the family's elders, who are the custodians of culture, decide based on their customs and culture. Several behaviors have been shown to prevent women from accessing prenatal care in a way that reduces their risk of maternal death [26].

3.2 Culture-related factors

Early marriage, genital mutilation, limited women's power in decision-making, cultural beliefs, and harmful traditional practices were identified to be the factors influencing maternal mortality under cultural factors [26, 30, 31]. The problems that cause maternal mortality have been shown to be influenced by customs or culturally relevant elements. In this context, women who participated in the research that are included stated that it is extremely difficult for them to decide to visit the healthcare facilities owing to culture because they are not permitted to make decisions [26, 28, 32]. The main factor in this theme was limited women's power in decision-making (n = 3, 43%), which means that elders are responsible for making decisions for pregnant women according to culture [26, 29]. Therefore, older women hold power over the outcomes of ANC attendance.

3.3 Pregnant-women-related factors

In this theme, the subthemes that were identified were: late ANC booking, frequency of ANC attendance, unwanted pregnancy, and lack of knowledge [26, 30, 31]. The studies revealed that married women attended ANC earlier than unmarried women. Moreover, employed women attended ANC most frequently compared to unemployed women. Moreover, it was found that most women visiting ANC had planned pregnancies rather than unintended pregnancies [30].

The review found that several pregnant women in the studies did not show up for ANC on time. Hence, insufficient ANC attendance or late reservations may prevent women from receiving a diagnosis for diseases that could arise early in

Themes	Subthemes
Community members' opinions about the state of maternal health	Lack of knowledge,
	Traditional birth attendance experience,
	Previous childbirth experience,
	Perceptions of risk
	And facility-based experiences
Culture-related factors	Early marriage
	Genital mutilation
	Limited women's power in decision-making
	Cultural beliefs
	Harmful traditional practices
Pregnant-women-related factors	Late ANC booking,
	Frequency of ANC attendance
	Unwanted pregnancy
	Lack of knowledge
Healthcare system factors	The distance where the healthcare facilities are situated
	Shortage of resources which also includes human resources,
	Provision of services only within the allocated hours
	Lack of privacy in the healthcare facilities
Choice of care	The attitude of healthcare practitioners in the healthcare facilities
	Past birth experiences
Traditional-birth-attendant-related factors	Poor referral practices for obstetric complications
	Poor relationships with the local healthcare team

Table 3.
Themes and subthemes.

pregnancy and result in complications that could result in maternal mortality [26, 30, 31]. Lack of awareness of the significance of attending antenatal clinics, unintended pregnancy, and unprofessional behavior of healthcare professionals all contributed to late booking.

3.4 Healthcare system factors

The healthcare system factors, such as distance from the healthcare facilities, a lack of resources, including human resources, the provision of services only during the designated hours, and a lack of privacy in the healthcare facilities, were also found to be contributing factors to maternal mortality [26, 30, 32, 33]. Lack of privacy discouraged pregnant women from going to the hospital; they claimed it was preferable to give birth in front of their husbands and family members than in front of medical personnel. Due to poor mobility, pregnant women who live in those areas are not frequently visited or attended by healthcare facilities [30, 32]. According to the literature, women are prevented from visiting medical facilities because; when they go for an ANC appointment, there is occasionally no medical personnel available to help them or, more frequently, there is no medical equipment available to offer them the necessary care [26, 30].

3.5 Choice of care

Pregnant women in this situation typically rely on TBAs for assistance rather than contact medical institutions [26, 29–33]. The included studies indicated that past delivery experiences and the attitudes of healthcare professionals in healthcare facilities are two factors that influence the choice of women. Past birth experiences in medical facilities accounted for most of the theme's variance (n = 6, 71%) [26, 29–33]. The ladies in the included studies stated that they were persuaded to avoid using healthcare facilities while pregnant by their unpleasant experiences there.

3.6 Traditional-birth-attendant-related factors

Poor referral procedures for maternal problems and strained relationships with the local medical staff were factors that were identified under this theme [27]. Because there is a dearth of referrals when there is an obstetric difficulty, there are no partnerships between healthcare facilities and traditional birth attendants, which exacerbates the issues that could cause maternal mortality. Traditional birth attendants have stated that traditional substances can be utilized to handle difficulties such as protracted labor, obstructed labor, retained placenta, and maternal bleeding instead of sending the women to a medical center [27]. The absence of referrals when issues develop has also been linked to a bad interaction between the TBAs and the neighborhood healthcare institutions [27].

The themes were conceptualized hereunder into a framework that provides the interrelationship triad between pregnant women, healthcare facilities, and traditional birth attendants. The review provided that both directions of the relationship triad have contributory factors at different levels (see **Figure 2**).

4. Discussion

In this systematic review, five major factors that influence maternal mortality in Africa emerged. These were identified as past birth delivery, late booking, lack of transportation to the facility, attitude of healthcare professionals, and traditional practices. According to the included studies, traditional practices are the major factor leading to complications causing maternal mortality. It has been revealed that TBAs do not refer pregnant women to healthcare facilities for further management. However, they report to the traditional authorities about the complications [27]. Poor referral systems between TBA and healthcare professionals are a serious concern as the two sectors should approach maternal care collaboratively, involving a positive combined effort to eradicate avoidable maternal mortality.

Although maternal mortality declines in developed countries, it remains unexpectedly high in rural communities. Various factors have been found to contribute to maternal mortality. The elements mentioned above had a significant role in this systematic study regarding problems resulting in maternal death. However, all the factors that affect maternal mortality are grouped under cultural norms and practices. The included research showed that culture has a big impact on expecting mothers.

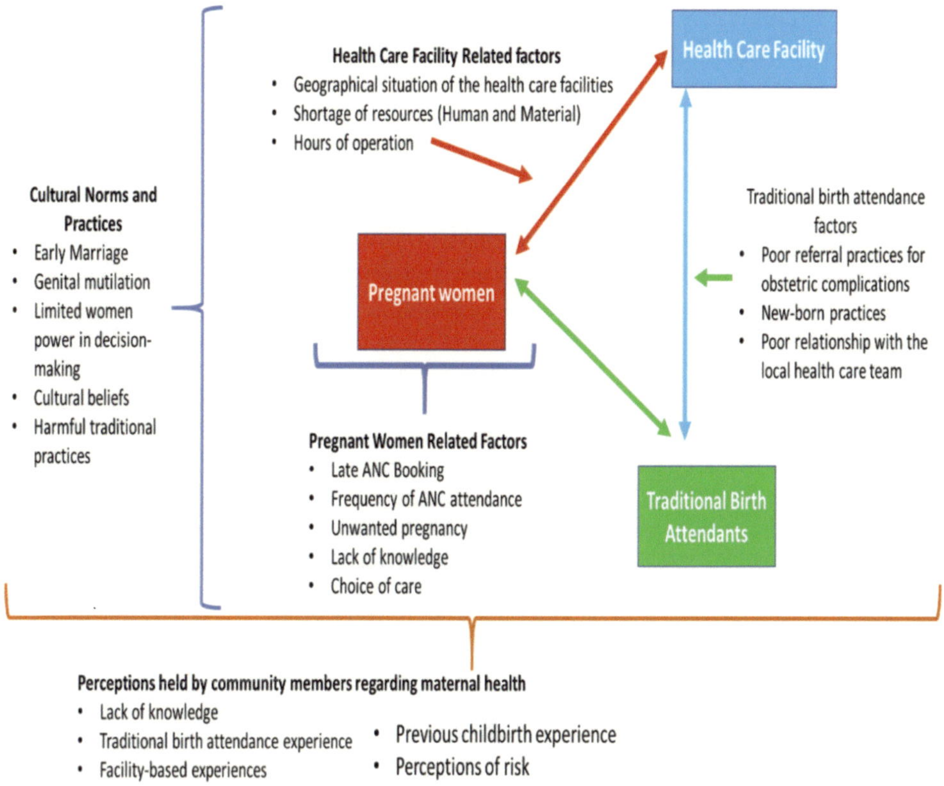

Figure 2.
Conceptual map of the systematic review results.

To avoid witchcraft and keep the baby from dying, some women, for example, choose not to enroll in ANC since the culture forbids them from being seen while pregnant. Many customs prevent women from seeking out healthcare facilities at this time. It has been noted that multifaceted factors heavily impact the goal of reducing maternal mortality. Thus, sociocultural factors have been reported to take the lead and warrant the collaborative approach from the health system and traditional or community-based stakeholders. Similar issues have been raised in Pakistan, and the most challenging struggle to reduce maternal mortality is firmly rooted in tackling sociocultural practices that build hindrances to maternal care-seeking [34, 35].

It is indeed difficult for African women to find themselves cornered between sociocultural practices that they have been taught from their initiation through rites of passage and the teachings from the healthcare professional in primary healthcare facilities. A need for a socioculturally congruent approach to creating awareness of the sociocultural maternal health practices' impact on their health has the potential to reduce maternal mortality. Community outreach programs are critical through community gatherings, door-to-door family-based visits, social media, and the use of community health workers can be implemented and maintained sustainably to help reduce maternal mortality. Some sociocultural factors are imposed based on the family history, knowledge, and beliefs, which becomes an internalized body of knowledge that requires combined effort to correct. There is also a need to eradicate the one-size-fits-all approach from TBAs, elderly family members, and traditional healthcare practitioners. This is important given that most women will still go through the cultural practice regardless of the previous encounter that may not have ended well.

Besides the sociocultural factors, the attitudes of healthcare professionals, mainly midwives, are reported to be a considerable challenge that also, in a way, influences women rather to follow cultural practices and continue to use TBA. There is a need for healthcare professionals to be capacitated in terms of positive values grounded by the Ubuntu philosophy. Thus, the ability to attend to pregnant women with respect, courtesy and all positive morals and within the positive boundaries of ethics. The latter is imperative and crucial as women need to rely on both systems for the greater good of the maternal care outcome.

5. Identified gaps

The reviewed research studies showed that culture is important, particularly for pregnant women, and that older persons are mostly in charge of maintaining it. Early booking is one of the strategies to reduce problems that can result in maternal death, according to the WHO [1]. But according to the research included, some women are forbidden from leaving the house when they are expecting to avoid witchcraft. Hence, sociocultural traditions and the health system's needs must be in harmony.

6. Conclusion

Globally, maternal mortality is a crucial issue. The millennium development goal (MDG) of 38 deaths per 10,000 live births was not achieved in 2015 due to several issues. This comprehensive review identifies the causes of maternal mortality in Africa. The interventions being developed are intended to lessen this issue and are also based on patient-reported barriers to attending ANC or maternity check-ups at healthcare facilities to avoid problems that could result in maternal mortality. Due to many traditional circumstances, there still appears to be a gap in the required compliance in other regions, particularly in rural areas. It is anticipated that relevant interventions that are collaborative can be created using the data from this review, which will assist in preventing the problems that cause maternal death and achieving SDG 3 target 1.

Acknowledgements

The authors acknowledge the University of Venda librarian for assistance in the literature search.

The authors also acknowledge SAMRC for funding this study.

Conflict of interest

The authors declare no conflict of interest.

Author details

Thendo Gertie Makhado[1]*, Lufuno Makhado[2], Mutshinyalo Lizzy Netshikeweta[1] and Azwidihwi Rose Tshililo[1]

1 Department of Advanced Nursing Sciences, University of Venda, South Africa

2 Office of the Executive Dean, University of Venda, South Africa

*Address all correspondence to: gertie.makhado@univen.ac.za

References

[1] World Health Organization. Maternal Health in Nigeria: Generating Information for Action. Geneva, Switzerland: World Health Organization; 2019. Available from: https://www.who.int/reproductivehealth/maternal-health-nigeria/en

[2] Piane GM. Maternal mortality in Nigeria: A literature review. World Medical & Health Policy. 2019;**11**(1):83-94

[3] Olonade O, Olawande TI, Alabi OJ, Imhonopi D. Maternal mortality and maternal health care in Nigeria: Implications for socio-economic development. Open access Macedonian Journal of Medical Sciences. 2019;**7**(5):849

[4] Meh C, Thind A, Ryan B, Terry A. Levels and determinants of maternal mortality in northern and southern Nigeria. BMC Pregnancy and Childbirth. 2019;**19**(1):1-3

[5] Batist J. An intersectional analysis of maternal mortality in sub-Saharan Africa: A human rights issue. Journal of Global Health. 2019;**9**(1):1-4

[6] Yemane Y, Tiruneh F. Incidence-proportion of maternal near-misses and associated factors in Southwest Ethiopia: A prospective cross-sectional study. International Journal of Women's Health. 2020;**12**:1125

[7] Ahinkorah BO, Ameyaw EK, Seidu AA, Odusina EK, Keetile M, Yaya S. Examining barriers to healthcare access and utilization of antenatal care services: Evidence from demographic health surveys in sub-Saharan Africa. BMC Health Services Research. 2021;**21**(1):1-6

[8] Cia U. Central Intelligence Agency-the World Factbook. New Zealand: Central Intelligence Agency; 2016

[9] Buor D, Bream K. An analysis of the determinants of maternal mortality in sub-Saharan Africa. Journal of Women's Health. 2004;**13**(8):926-938

[10] Adde KS, Dickson KS, Amu H. Prevalence and determinants of the place of delivery among reproductive age women in sub–Saharan Africa. PLoS One. 2020;**15**(12):e0244875

[11] Lancaster L, Barnes RF, Correia M, Luis E, Boaventura I, Silva P, et al. Maternal death and postpartum hemorrhage in sub-Saharan Africa–a pilot study in metropolitan Mozambique. Research and Practice in Thrombosis and Haemostasis. 2020;**4**(3):402-412

[12] Van Malderen C, Amouzou A, Barros AJ, Masquelier B, Van Oyen H, Speybroeck N. Socioeconomic factors contributing to under-five mortality in sub-Saharan Africa: A decomposition analysis. BMC Public Health. 2019;**19**(1):1-9

[13] Mumtaz S, Bahk J, Khang YH. Current status and determinants of maternal healthcare utilization in Afghanistan: Analysis from Afghanistan demographic and health survey 2015. PLoS One. 2019;**14**(6):e0217827

[14] Tuyisenge G, Hategeka C, Kasine Y, Luginaah I, Cechetto D, Rulisa S. Mothers' perceptions and experiences of using maternal healthcare services in Rwanda. Women & Health. 2019;**59**(1):68-84

[15] Jolivet RR, Moran AC, O'Connor M, Chou D, Bhardwaj N, Newby H, et al. Ending preventable maternal mortality: Phase II of a multi-step process to develop a monitoring framework, 2016-2030. BMC Pregnancy and Childbirth. 2018;**18**(1):1-3

[16] Moodley J, Fawcus S, Pattinson R. Improvements in maternal mortality in South Africa. South African Medical Journal. 2018;**108**(3):4-8

[17] Creanga AA. Maternal mortality in the United States: A review of contemporary data and their limitations. Clinical Obstetrics and Gynecology. 2018;**61**(2):296-306

[18] Bomela NJ. Maternal mortality by socio-demographic characteristics and cause of death in South Africa: 2007-2015. BMC Public Health. 2020;**20**(1):1-20

[19] Rahman MA, Halder HR, Islam SM. Effects of COVID-19 on maternal institutional delivery: Fear of a rise in maternal mortality. Journal of Global Health. 2021:**11**

[20] Gulumser C, Engin-Ustun Y, Keskin L, Celen S, Sanisoglu S, Karaahmetoglu S, et al. Maternal mortality due to hemorrhage: Population-based study in Turkey. The Journal of Maternal-Fetal & Neonatal Medicine. 2019;**32**(23):3998-4004

[21] Say L, Chou D, Gemmill A, Tunçalp Ö, Moller AB, Daniels J, et al. Global causes of maternal death: A WHO systematic analysis. The Lancet Global Health. 2014;**2**(6):e323-e333

[22] Ariyo O, Ozodiegwu ID, Doctor HV. The influence of the social and cultural environment on maternal mortality in Nigeria: Evidence from the 2013 demographic and health survey. PLoS One. 2017;**12**(12):e0190285

[23] Yarney L. Does knowledge on sociocultural factors associated with maternal mortality affect maternal health decisions? A cross-sectional study of the Greater Accra region of Ghana. BMC Pregnancy and Childbirth. 2019;**19**(1):1-2

[24] Aborigo RA, Reidpath DD, Oduro AR, Allotey P. Male involvement in maternal health: Perspectives of opinion leaders. BMC Pregnancy and Childbirth. 2018;**18**(1):1-0

[25] Moher D, Liberati A, Tetzlaff J, Altman DG, Altman D, Antes G, et al. Preferred reporting items for systematic reviews and meta-analyses: The PRISMA statement (Chinese edition). Journal of Chinese Integrative Medicine. 2009;**7**(9):889-896

[26] Kea AZ, Tulloch O, Datiko DG, Theobald S, Kok MC. Exploring barriers to the use of formal maternal health services and priority areas for action in Sidama zone, southern Ethiopia. BMC Pregnancy and Childbirth. 2018;**18**(1):1-2

[27] Bucher S, Konana O, Liechty E, Garces A, Gisore P, Marete I, et al. Self-reported practices among traditional birth attendants surveyed in western Kenya: A descriptive study. BMC Pregnancy and Childbirth. 2016;**16**(1):1-7

[28] Berhan Y, Berhan A. Reasons for persistently high maternal and perinatal mortalities in Ethiopia: Part II-socio-economic and cultural factors. Ethiopian Journal of Health Sciences. 2014;**24**:119-136

[29] Abubakar R, Yohanna S, Zubairu H. Influence of health decision making on maternal complications among women delivered at a general hospital, North-Western Nigeria. Nigerian journal of clinical practice. 2020;**23**(5):675-679

[30] Sibiya MN, Ngxongo TS, Bhengu TJ. Access and utilization of antenatal care services in a rural community of eThekwini district in KwaZulu-Natal. International Journal of Africa Nursing Sciences. 2018;**8**:1-7

[31] Muhwava LS, Morojele N, London L. Psychosocial factors associated with early initiation and frequency of antenatal care (ANC) visits in a rural and urban setting in South Africa: A cross-sectional survey. BMC Pregnancy and Childbirth. 2016;**16**(1):1-9

[32] Marchie CL. Sociocultural factors as correlates of maternal mortality in Edo south Senatorial District, Nigerai. Asian Pacific Journal of Reproduction. 2012;**1**(4):315-317

[33] Ansong J, Asampong E, Adongo PB. Sociocultural beliefs and practices during pregnancy, child birth, and postnatal period: A qualitative study in southern Ghana. Cogent Public Health. 2022;**9**(1):2046908

[34] Omer S, Zakar R, Zakar MZ, Fischer F. The influence of social and cultural practices on maternal mortality: A qualitative study from South Punjab, Pakistan. Reproductive Health. 2021;**18**(1):1-2. DOI: 10.1186/s12978-021-01151-6

[35] Sumankuuro J, Crockett J, Wang S. Maternal health care initiatives: Causes of morbidities and mortalities in two rural districts of upper west region, Ghana. PLoS One. 2017;**12**(8):e0183644

Section 4

Different Approach to Family Planning

Chapter 7

Male Involvement in Family Planning Services

Mesfin Abebe, Tsion Mulat Tebeje, Wondwosen Molla and Getnet Melaku

Abstract

Family planning is the ability of individuals and couples to anticipate and obtain their preferred number of children, spacing, and timing of births. It is accomplished through the use of contraceptive methods and the treatment of involuntary infertility. Family planning is important for the well-being of women and their families, and it can help a country reduce poverty and achieve the SDGs faster. When family planning methods are used effectively, they assist couples in having the number of children they desire, improve maternal and child health, which may assist women in avoiding unintended pregnancies, and lower risk factors for maternal and child mortality. Increasing the use of condoms and vasectomies among men is only one aspect of male involvement in family planning. It also includes the number of men who support and encourage their partners and peers to use family planning, as well as the number of men who influence policy to make it more favorable to promoting male-related programs. Men's participation is critical to women's health and program completion, as it promotes shared responsibility for birth control, contraceptive reputation, and thus the women are more likely to adopt and continue using beginning prevention if their partner's active assistance.

Keywords: male involvement, family planning, magnitude, associated factors, Ethiopia

1. Introduction

Family planning is the process by which individuals and couples predict and achieve the number, spacing, and timing of children they desire. By using contraceptive methods and treating unintentional infertility, it is achieved [1, 2]. It encompasses the services, policies, information, attitudes, practices, and commodities, such as contraception, that enable women, men, couples, and adolescents to avoid unintended pregnancy and make decisions about whether and/or when to have a child [3]. Programs for family planning (FP) have mainly focused on women. However, there is a shift to involve men in supporting and using FP services as a result of the focus on gender equity for best health. The World Health Organization (WHO) and the Ministry of Health in the majority of countries have recommended and approved the use of FP methods as an effective intervention, and men, as the decision-makers in most African families, have a crucial role to play in this process [4].

Family planning has been a major concern in programs to reduce the population as well as those that promote and improve reproductive health [5]. Family planning is critical for the health of women and families, and it can accelerate a country's progress toward eradicating poverty and achieving the Sustainable Development Goals. Effective family planning techniques enable couples to have as many children as they want, improve maternal and child health, which may assist women in avoiding unintended pregnancies, and reduce risk factors for maternal and infant mortality [6].

The use of contraception has been linked to decreased fertility, better maternal and child health due to birth spacing and fewer pregnancies, and increased women's empowerment by enabling them to complete their education and enter the workforce [7] . The two types of contraceptive methods. This are modern and traditional methods of contraceptive. Male and female sterilization, IUDs, implants, injectable contraceptives, pills, male and female condoms, emergency contraception, and the lactational amenorrhea method are all modern methods. (LAM), While traditional methods consist of rhythm (calendar), withdrawal, and folk methods [8, 9].

Contraception has a number of advantages, including ensuring couples have the number of children they want and lowering infant, perinatal, and maternal mortality. Additionally, it lowers the chance of HIV transmission, STI acquisition, and unintended pregnancy. Furthermore, it reduces pregnancy and birth-related complications by giving a mother enough time to recover from previous pregnancy complications [8]. Globally, women have played a significant role in household management and decision-making regarding their own health care and life through family planning. There has been a significant improvement in family planning utilization and birth rates. However, male involvement in family planning remains minimal, with men playing a secondary role [10].

Male involvement in family planning (FP) refers to all organizational actions aimed at increasing the acceptability and uptake of FP among both sexes. It includes men participating in decision making, approving it, or encouraging their spouse's use of family planning [11]. Through increased spousal communication, male involvement can lead to contraceptive use [12–14]. It encompasses more than just an increase in the proportion of men who use condoms and get vasectomies. It also includes the proportion of men who support and encourage their partners and their peers to use FP and who influence public policy to make male-related programs more widely promoted. In this context, "male involvement" refers to activities aimed at men as a distinct group with the goal of raising couples' acceptance and use of family planning, more so than male contraception [15].

In African nations, men are frequently the main decision-makers, and this has a big impact on their spouse's health and access to healthcare, including decisions about family planning (FP) [16]. Family planning is critical for slowing unsustainable population growth and its negative effects on the economy, environment, and national and regional development efforts [9]. Men are also blamed for a large proportion of their female partners' poor reproductive health. Furthermore, male involvement aids not only in the acceptance of a contraceptive but also in its effective use and continuation [9].

Family planning is crucial for achieving the goals and the post-2015 development agenda. The five SDG themes of People, Planet, Prosperity, Peace, and Partnership can all advance more quickly as a result. In the time frame of the SDGs, there is a chance for the world to achieve significant convergence between the developed and developing worlds, ending avoidable child and maternal deaths and achieving relative parity in addressing the family planning requirements of women, men, couples, and teenagers who want to space or limit childbearing [3]. Target 3.7 of the Sustainable Development Goals (SDGs) calls for universal access to sexual and reproductive health care services, including birth control, information, and education, by the end of 2030, and thus the integration of reproductive health into national strategy and programs [1, 17, 18]. Men's involvement in reproductive health issues is essential for achieving the SDGs. Furthermore, increasing economic development requires regulating fertility to the level of substitution. Family planning can reduce maternal and child mortality by 32% and 10%, respectively [19]. Male participation includes not only male contraception but also all other national program activities aimed at increasing male awareness, acceptability, and prevalence of family planning methods. The primary goal of family planning is to allow women and men to plan their families and space their children using modern contraceptives [20]. Sub-Saharan Africa has the highest fertility rate (more than 5 children per woman) as well as the fastest growth rate (on average 2.5 percent per year) [21].

According to UN projections, the population of Sub-Saharan Africa will reach 2.12 billion by 2050 [22]. The second-most populous country in Africa is Ethiopia. It has the highest rate of annual growth (2.6%), infant mortality (43/1000 live births), and maternal mortality (412 per 100,000 live births) [23, 24]. Over the previous ten years, the Ethiopian population increased, rising from 55.18 million in 1994 to 112 million in 2019 and probably over 114 million in 2020 [22]. The United Nations reported that in 2019 Africa had a contraceptive prevalence rate (CPR) of 29.4%, sub-Saharan Africa had a CPR of 28.5%, Ethiopia had a CPR of 26.5%, and there was a 22% unmet need for FP in Africa [1]. According to the EDHS 2019 report, usage of modern contraceptives among married women has increased since 2000, 2005, 2011, 2016, and 2019 by 6%, 14%, 27%, 35%, and 41%, respectively, while usage of traditional methods has remained stable for the years of 2005, 2011, 2016, and 2019 at about 1%. Injectable usage among modern methods of contraception, which increased steadily from 3% in 2000 to 27% in 2019, and primarily to blame for the rise in the use of modern methods than others [24].

Studies have shown that the involvement of men significantly changed the way family planning is used in many developing nations. Their participation in using family planning services is still minimal. Several studies on male involvement in family planning use and reproductive health have been carried out in Ethiopia in various regions of the nation. The husband plays a significant role in this country in approving or disapproving the use of family planning services by their wives based on a number of barriers between these religions and cultures that are said to have a negative impact on them. This is due to the fact that in many developing nations, such as Ethiopia, men frequently have the deciding influence over major family decisions, such as their wives' use of contraceptives [25].

Traditionally, men have been excluded from receiving or providing information about sexuality, reproductive health, and birth spacing. They have also been ignored or excluded in some way from participating in many family planning programs, owing to the perception that family planning is a woman's domain [14, 26]. To reduce contraceptive discontinuation rates, male participation is required [27]. In Ethiopia the extent of male involvement in family planning service utilization 68% from a previous study [28]. Few pieces of research suggest that male involvement can increase uptake and continuation of family planning methods by improving spousal communication through pathways of increased knowledge or decreased male opposition [12, 13] . Husbands have a significant impact on women's access to family planning services and other forms of healthcare [29].

2. Factors affecting male involvement in family planning

Studies done in African contexts have found that men's lack of knowledge about contraceptive methods, as well as gender norms regarding men's roles, may be important factors in men's negative perceptions of and disengagement from family planning. Some studies also suggest that spousal communication is low even in situations where men approve of contraceptive methods [30, 31]. The West African Demographic and Health Survey found that about 75% of men and women had not discussed family planning with their partners in the year before the survey [32]. In Tanzania, 45% of married women said they were unaware of their husbands' thoughts on family planning or thought they were opposed to it, even though in fact many of the husbands were in favor [33]. Several socioeconomic factors, including religion and tradition, the role of women in decision-making in society, cultural values, and others, have a significant impact on family planning services in Ethiopia. Women's access to family planning services may be impacted by their status in the family, the economy, and public life [34].

In a study conducted in Kenya, it was discovered that male involvement in family planning was significantly associated with demographic factors such as age, the number of children, educational attainment, and social factors such as social group membership and religion of the respondent. Knowing a place that provides family planning services, having a general understanding of family planning, and being aware of particular family planning techniques accessible to both men and women were all significantly associated. However, only the ease of access to family planning services for men was found to be strongly associated with male participation [26].

Another Nigerian study found that the level of education, the number of living children, and approval of family planning are all indicators of male involvement in reproductive health care [35]. According to a Bangladesh study, the level of male involvement was associated to schooling experience, type of residency, and exposure to electronic media [36]. Men who participate in family planning, in addition to using contraception, support and encourage their partners' contraceptive needs and decisions, encourage their peers to use contraception, and influence public policy to improve male-related programs [37]. One of the essential health care services that can promote and ensure reproductive health is family planning. According to studies, males' intentions to discuss family planning are influenced by their attitudes, norms, and self-efficacy. Males' perceptions of family planning as a female responsibility also influence family planning [20].

In many sub-Saharan African nations, men were also key decision-makers in the household and typically opposed their partners' use of contraceptives. The male predominance in decision-making among couples and its impact on women's decision-making power in the use of contraceptives are both caused by women's young age at marriage, the age gap between husband and wife, polygamous family structures, and culture. Decisions about limiting fertility are made by the husband or his parents in societies where gender stratification is common [38, 39].

Recently, the husband's involvement in the decision-making process for family planning has come to light as an important factor influencing the use of contraceptives. Men who participate in family planning make decisions about using contraception [12], but study indicates that male involvement is lower in less developed nations [40, 41].

Research from the past suggested that men should even participate in family planning programs [41], but until now, the majority of countries worldwide have only targeted women in these programs [42, 43]. According to some studies, men as well as women must be involved in order for targeted family planning coverage to be successfully achieved [44]. According to study done in Malawi, targeting men for family planning interventions may greatly increase the uptake of contraceptives [45]. Others suggested that targeting both spouses with family planning education rather than focusing solely on one gender might be more effective [46]. t has also been demonstrated how important it is to involve husbands in family planning initiatives in order to increase the use of modern contraceptives rather than traditional methods [47].

Men typically serve as the health care system's gatekeepers in developing countries. They are the ones who make the majority of decisions that have a direct impact on the health of their spouse and their children. Their choices have an impact on resource utilization, access to health care services, contraceptive use, birth spacing, the availability of nutritious food, and the workload of women [48].

However, research on couples' contraceptive use has primarily focused on the knowledge, attitudes, discussion, and intentions regarding family planning rather than examining the specific effects of programs on the use of contraceptives and family planning services [49]. In order to achieve higher levels of contraceptive prevalence, efforts must be made to promote spousal cooperation and communication as well as to encourage men's involvement in family planning [44].

According to a qualitative study conducted in Nepal, men's education and attitude, knowledge and awareness, sociocultural factors, psychological factors, aspects of the health system, and policies all have a significant impact on male involvement in reproductive health [48]. Another study done in Ethiopia found that lack of knowledge, myths, misconceptions, access issues, the desire to have more children, fear of social rejection, concerns about side effects, the husband's opposition and religious prohibition, negative attitudes, the husband and partner's educational status, the number of living children, the male approach to family planning, male family planning awareness, and conversation with the wife about family planning have all contributed to the lack of access to family planning services [21, 27, 50–52].

3. Conclusion

Men's involvement in family planning could increase the prevalence of contraception in a number of ways, including by giving couples who are dissatisfied with their current method options, increasing male contraceptive use, encouraging more conversation between sexual partners, and altering male attitudes toward contraception. According to a study conducted in Ethiopia, husband participation in home visits during discussions increased the likelihood that couples would start using contraceptives and keep using them [34].

Author details

Mesfin Abebe[1*], Tsion Mulat Tebeje[2], Wondwosen Molla[1] and Getnet Melaku[1]

1 Department of Midwifery, College of Medicine and Health Science, Dilla University, Dilla, Ethiopia

2 School of Public Health, College of Medicine and Health Science, Dilla University, Dilla, Ethiopia

*Address all correspondence to: mesfiaau@gmail.com; mesfin.abebe@du.edu.et

References

[1] Organization WH. Family Planning/ Contraception: Fact Sheet. WHO 2017; 2018

[2] Gonie A, Wudneh A, Nigatu D, Dendir Z. Determinants of family planning use among married women in bale eco-region, Southeast Ethiopia: A community based study. BMC Women's Health. 2018;**18**(1):1-10

[3] Starbird E, Norton M, Marcus R. Investing in family planning: Key to achieving the sustainable development goals. Global Health: Science and Practice. 2016;**4**(2):191-210

[4] Amuzie CI, Nwamoh UN, Ukegbu A, Umeokonkwo CD, Azuogu BN, Agbo UO, et al. Determinants of male involvement in family planning services in Abia State, Southeast Nigeria. Contraception and Reproductive Medicine. 2022;**7**(1):1-9

[5] Kleinman RL, Senanayake P. Family Planning: Meeting Challenges, Promoting Choices. CRC Press; 1993

[6] Ewunetie GE, Alemu MD, Chanie MG. Why modern family planning needs of women is not met in South Gondar zone, Ethiopia? PLOS Global Public Health. 2022;**2**(6):e0000335

[7] Al Riyami A, Afifi M, Mabry RM. Women's autonomy, education and employment in Oman and their influence on contraceptive use. Reproductive Health Matters. 2004;**12**(23):144-154

[8] Mulatu T, Sintayehu Y, Dessie Y, Deressa M. Modern family planning utilization and its associated factors among currently married women in rural eastern Ethiopia: A community-based study. BioMed research international. 29 Dec 2020;**13**(20):150-165

[9] Adera A, Belete T, Gebru A, Hagos A, Gebregziabher W. Assessment of the role of men in family planning utilization at Edaga-Hamuse town, Tigray, North Ethiopia. American Journal of Nursing Science. 2015;**4**(4):174

[10] Mercy Nwankwo C, Immaculate O. Factors influencing male involvement in family planning among married couples seeking maternity and pediatric services in Chuk. 2022 (unpublished research)

[11] Mulatu T, Sintayehu Y, Dessie Y, Dheresa M. Male involvement in family planning use and associated factors among currently married men in rural eastern Ethiopia. SAGE Open Medicine. 2022;**10**:20503121221094178

[12] Kabagenyi A, Jennings L, Reid A, Nalwadda G, Ntozi J, Atuyambe L. Barriers to male involvement in contraceptive uptake and reproductive health services: A qualitative study of men and women's perceptions in two rural districts in Uganda. Reproductive Health. 2014;**11**(1):1-9

[13] Hartmann M, Gilles K, Shattuck D, Kerner B, Guest G. Changes in couples' communication as a result of a male-involvement family planning intervention. Journal of Health Communication. 2012;**17**(7):802-819

[14] Adelekan A, Omoregie P, Edoni E. Male involvement in family planning: Challenges and way forward. International Journal of Population Research. 2014;**2014**:1-10

[15] Walle Y, Alamrew Z. The current states of male involvement on family

planning and factors correlated with among male factory workers in Bahir Dar City. American Journal of Public Health Research. 2014;**2**(5):188-197

[16] Namee Wambete S, Baru A, Serwaa D, Kojo Dzantor E, Poku-Agyemang E, Wekem Kukeba M, et al. Attitude of Reproductive Age Women towards Male Involvement in Family Planning; a Community-Based Cross-Sectional Study in Nakawa Division. Kampala, Uganda: medRxiv; 2022 2022.07. 14.22277630

[17] Kantorová V, Wheldon MC, Dasgupta AN, Ueffing P, Castanheira HC. Contraceptive use and needs among adolescent women aged 15-19: Regional and global estimates and projections from 1990 to 2030 from a Bayesian hierarchical modelling study. PLoS One. 2021;**16**(3):e0247479

[18] SDG U. Sustainable development goals. The energy progress report Tracking SDG. 2019;7

[19] Anbesu EW, Aychiluhm SB, Kahsay ZH. Male involvement in family planning use and its determinants in Ethiopia: A systematic review and meta-analysis protocol. Systematic Reviews. 2022;**11**(1):19. DOI: 10.1186/s13643-022-01891-x

[20] Parija PP, Pal A, Panigrahi SK, Thakur P, Pal R. Male involvement in family planning in a rural area of India. Journal of Family Medicine and Primary Care. 2022;**11**(5):1943

[21] Abose A, Adhena G, Dessie Y. Assessment of male involvement in long-acting and permanent contraceptive use of their partner in west Badewacho, southern Ethiopia. Open Access Journal of Contraception. 2021;**12**:63-72

[22] Nation U. World Population Prospect 2019. New York, NY, USA: Department of Economic and Social Affairs, Population Division; 2019

[23] CSA I. Central Statistical Agency. Ethiopia Demographic and Health Survey. 2016

[24] Central S, Program T, ICF Rockville M. Ethiopia mini Demographic and Health Survey. Ethiopia USA: Central Statistical Agency Addis Ababa; 2019

[25] Assefa L, Shasho Z, Kasaye HK, Tesa E, Turi E, Fekadu G. Men's involvement in family planning service utilization among married men in Kondala district, western Ethiopia: A community-based comparative cross-sectional study. Contraception and Reproductive Medicine. 2021;**6**(1):16. DOI: 10.1186/s40834-021-00160-x

[26] Butto D, Mburu S. Factors associated with male involvement in family planning in West Pokot County, Kenya. Universal Journal of Public Health. 2015;**3**(4):160-168

[27] Wondim G, Degu G, Teka Y, Diress G. Male involvement in family planning utilization and associated factors in Womberma District, northern Ethiopia: Community-based cross-sectional study. Open Access Journal of Contraception. 2020;**11**:197

[28] Kejela G, Mira G, Gaga B, Muktar A, Ololo B, Bezabehe S. The role of male involvement in modern family planning utilization and associated factors in Arba Minch town, Gamo Gofa zone, Ethiopia. European Journal of Preventive Medicine. 2017;**5**:39

[29] Chekole MK, Kahsay ZH, Medhanyie AA, Gebreslassie MA, Bezabh AM. Husbands' involvement in family planning use and its associated

factors in pastoralist communities of Afar, Ethiopia. Reproductive Health. 2019;**16**:1-7

[30] Onyango MA, Owoko S, Oguttu M. Factors that influence male involvement in sexual and reproductive health in western Kenya: A qualitative study. African Journal of Reproductive Health. 2010;**14**(4):43-55

[31] Nalwadda G, Mirembe F, Byamugisha J, Faxelid E. Persistent high fertility in Uganda: Young people recount obstacles and enabling factors to use of contraceptives. BMC Public Health. 2010;**10**(1):1-13

[32] Ezeh AC, Seroussi M, Raggers H. Men's Fertility, Contraceptive Use, and Reproductive Preferences. Macro International; 1996

[33] Toure L. Male Involvement in Family Planning: A Review of Programmes and Selected Programme Initiatives in Africa. 1996

[34] Terefe A, Larson CP. Modern contraception use in Ethiopia: Does involving husbands make a difference? American Journal of Public Health. 1993;**83**(11):1567-1571

[35] Ani F, Abiodun O, Sotunsa J, Faturoti O, Imaralu J, Olaleye A. Demographic factors related to male involvement in reproductive health care services in Nigeria. The European Journal of Contraception & Reproductive Health Care. 2016;**21**(1):57-67

[36] Bishwajit G, Tang S, Yaya S, Ide S, Fu H, Wang M, et al. Factors associated with male involvement in reproductive care in Bangladesh. BMC Public Health. 2017;**17**(1):1-8

[37] Kassa BG, Tenaw LA, Ayele AD, Tiruneh GA. Prevalence and determinants of the involvement of married men in family planning services in Ethiopia: A systematic review and meta-analysis. Women's Health. 2022;**18**:17455057221099083

[38] Hogan DP, Berhanu B, Hailemariam A. Household organization, women's autonomy, and contraceptive behavior in southern Ethiopia. Studies in Family Planning. 1999;**30**(4):302-314

[39] Bogale B, Wondafrash M, Tilahun T, Girma E. Married women's decision making power on modern contraceptive use in urban and rural southern Ethiopia. BMC Public Health 2011;**11**(1):1-7

[40] Ijadunola MY, Abiona TC, Ijadunola KT, Afolabi OT, Esimai OA, OlaOlorun FM. Male involvement in family planning decision making in Ile-Ife, Osun state, Nigeria. African Journal of Reproductive Health. 2010;**14**(4):43-55

[41] Sharma A. Male involvement in reproductive health: Women's perspective. Journal of Family Welfare. 2003;**49**:1-9

[42] Mekonnen W, Worku A. Determinants of low family planning use and high unmet need in Butajira District, south Central Ethiopia. Reproductive Health. 2011;**8**:1-8

[43] Abraham W, Adamu A, Deresse D. The involvement of men in family planning an application of transtheoretical model in Wolaita Soddo town South Ethiopia. Asian Journal of Medical Sciences. 2010;**2**(2):44-50

[44] Adugnaw B, Sibhatu B, Alemayehu A, Sudhakar M, Alemayehu B, Kebede D. Men's knowledge and spousal communication about modern family planning methods in Ethiopia. African Journal of Reproductive Health. 2011;**15**(4):24-32

[45] Shattuck D, Kerner B, Gilles K, Hartmann M, Ng'ombe T, Guest G. Encouraging contraceptive uptake by motivating men to communicate about family planning: The Malawi male motivator project. American Journal of Public Health. 2011;**101**(6):1089-1095

[46] Özgür S, Bozkurt AI, Özçirpici B. The effects of family planning education provided to different gender groups. BJOG: An International Journal of Obstetrics & Gynaecology. 2000;**107**(10):1226-1232

[47] Organization WH. Optimizing the Health Workforce for Effective Family Planning Services: Policy Brief. World Health Organization; 2012

[48] Sharma S, Kc B, Khatri A. Factors influencing male participation in reproductive health: A qualitative study. Journal of Multidisciplinary Healthcare. 2018;**11**:601-608

[49] Mwaikambo L, Speizer IS, Schurmann A, Morgan G, Fikree F. What works in family planning interventions: A systematic review. Studies in Family Planning. 2011;**42**(2):67-82

[50] Kassa M, Abajobir AA, Gedefaw M. Level of male involvement and associated factors in family planning services utilization among married men in Debremarkos town, Northwest Ethiopia. BMC International Health and Human Rights. 2014;**14**:1-8

[51] Gebremariam A, Addissie A. Knowledge and perception on long acting and permanent contraceptive methods in Adigrat town, Tigray, northern Ethiopia: A qualitative study. International Journal of Family Medicine. 2014;**20**

[52] Geltore TE, Lakew YY. Prevalence of male participation in modern contraceptive use among married men in Durame town southern Ethiopia: A community based cross sectional study, 2021. The Pan African Medical Journal. 2022:41